Veterinary Science and Medicine

Veterinary Science and Medicine

Aston Gunn

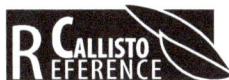

R CALLISTO REFERENCE

www.callistoreference.com

Callisto Reference,
118-35 Queens Blvd., Suite 400,
Forest Hills, NY 11375, USA

Visit us on the World Wide Web at:
www.callistoreference.com

ISBN: 978-1-64116-641-6 (Hardback)

Cataloging-in-Publication Data

Veterinary science and medicine / Aston Gunn.
       p. cm.
Includes bibliographical references and index.
ISBN 978-1-64116-641-6
1. Veterinary medicine. 2. Animals--Diseases. 3. Animal health. I. Gunn, Aston.
SF745 .V48 2022
636.089--dc23

Table of Contents

This book is a culmination of my many years of practice in this field. I attribute the success of this book to my support group. I would like to thank my parents who have showered me with unconditional love and support and my peers and professors for their constant guidance.

The branch of medicine which deals with the diagnosis, treatment and prevention of diseases and disorders in animals is referred to as veterinary science and medicine. It focuses on all species of animals as well as the conditions that affect them. Veterinary science also plays an important role in ensuring human health. This is done by preventing humans from getting infected by zoonotic diseases. Veterinary medicine also takes care of food safety and helps to maintain food supply by the monitoring and treatment of livestock health. This book is compiled in such a manner, that it will provide in-depth knowledge about the theory and practice of veterinary science and medicine. While understanding the long-term perspectives of the topics, it makes an effort in highlighting their impact as a modern tool for the growth of the discipline. The book, with its detailed analyses and data, will prove immensely beneficial to professionals and students involved in this area at various levels.

The details of chapters are provided below for a progressive learning:

Chapter – Introduction to Veterinary Science and Medicine

The branch of science which is centered on providing care to all animals is known as veterinary science. Veterinary medicine is a branch of medicine and veterinary science which focuses on the diagnosis, prevention and treatment of diseases in different families of animals. All the diverse principles of veterinary science and veterinary medicine have been carefully analyzed in this chapter.

Chapter – Animal Diseases and their Prevention

An animal disease can be defined as any impairment which hinders the normal functioning of an animal or its vital functions. Some of the diseases which can affect different animals are pseudorabies, equine viral arteritis, bird flu, rift valley fever and infectious bursal disease. This chapter has been carefully written to provide an easy understanding of these animal diseases as well as how they can be prevented.

Chapter – Zoonotic Diseases

The infectious diseases which spread from animals to humans are known as zoonotic diseases. They can be caused due to bacteria, viruses or parasites. Some of the common zoonotic diseases are anthrax, Ebola virus disease, rat-bite fever and rabies. This chapter closely examines these zoonotic diseases to provide an extensive understanding of the subject.

Chapter – Veterinary Practices and Surgical Procedures

Veterinary surgery is broadly classified into three categories, soft-tissue surgery, orthopedics and neurosurgery. Some of the common surgical procedures which are conducted on animals are onychectomy, devocalization, docking, urethrostomy and triple tibial osteotomy. The chapter closely examines these surgical practices to provide an extensive understanding of the subject.

Chapter – Veterinary Vaccines and Drugs

Veterinary vaccines and drugs play a major role in promoting animal health and reducing animal suffering. Some of the common veterinary vaccines are clostridial vaccine, DA2PPC vaccine and rabies vaccine. There are a number of drugs which are used to treat different ailments in animals. A few of them are acepromazine, boldenone and butorphanol. The diverse applications of these drugs and vaccines have been thoroughly discussed in this chapter.

Chapter – Alternative Veterinary Medicine

The use of alternative medicine for the treatment of animals is known as alternative veterinary medicine. A few branches of alternative veterinary medicine are veterinary acupuncture, ethnoveterinary medicine and veterinary chiropractic. The topics elaborated in this chapter will help in gaining a better perspective about these branches of alternative veterinary medicine.

Aston Gunn

1

Introduction to Veterinary Science and Medicine

The branch of science which is centered on providing care to all animals is known as veterinary science. Veterinary medicine is a branch of medicine and veterinary science which focuses on the diagnosis, prevention and treatment of diseases in different families of animals. All the diverse principles of veterinary science and veterinary medicine have been carefully analyzed in this chapter.

Veterinary Science

Just like people, animals get sick sometimes. As a result, there is a field of animal science devoted to caring for all species called Veterinary Science. A veterinarian (sometimes called a vet) is a doctor who works with all types of animals from dogs and cats to cows and sheep, and sometimes even animals like kangaroos! Veterinarians who only work with animals like dogs and cats are known as "small animal vets." Veterinarians who work with animals like cows, sheep, and pigs (livestock) are referred to as "large animal veterinarians. Veterinarians can also specialize in what is considered "exotic" animals like lizards and birds.

A veterinarian can work at an animal clinic. These offices are very similar to a human doctor's office, but vets have some special tools to examine their animal patients better. People can take their animals to the vet for just a check-up, but in special cases for other treatments and surgeries.

A large number of vet clinics offer mobile veterinary care services for farmers. These services are used in emergencies or when it is impractical to take an animal to the vet's office. For example, it is not practical to transport a cow to a vet's office when the cow is giving birth. Instead, the vet will visit the farm and help the cow there. Some livestock farms are so huge that they require a resident veterinarian to care for their animals. A resident veterinarian may live on site and care only for that farm's animals, or a vet might live locally and only work with certain farms in that area.

Currently, there are 22 different veterinary specialty organizations. These are specific skills area that a veterinarian has decided to dedicate their efforts to. Some of these specialties include behavior, dermatology, and anesthesia. To be a veterinary specialist, one must continue their education and complete more training. Following this they must pass a test about their specialty.

Some veterinarians specialize in pathology and work for diagnostic laboratories. These vets use special equipment to perform biopsies. A biopsy is the surgical removal and examination of tissue obtained from a living animal. Tissues make up the body. Tissues make up everything, even the bones, muscles, and blood. All types of veterinarians send in tissues to be tested, and the diagnostic veterinarians determine whether or not that animal has a disease and sends the results back.

Veterinary Medicine

Veterinary medicine, also called veterinary science is the medical specialty concerned with the prevention, control, diagnosis, and treatment of diseases affecting the health of domestic and wild animals and with the prevention of transmission of animal diseases to people. Veterinarians ensure a safe food supply for people by monitoring and maintaining the health of food-producing animals.

Persons serving as doctors to animals have existed since the earliest recorded times, and veterinary practice was already established as a specialty as early as 2000 BCE in Babylonia and Egypt. The ancient Greeks had a class of physicians who were called "horse-doctors," and the Latin term for the specialty, veterinarius ("pertaining to beast of burden"), came to denote the field in modern times. Today veterinarians serve worldwide in private and corporate clinical practice, academic programs, private industry, government service, public health, and military services. They often are supported in their work by other veterinary medicine professionals, such as veterinary nurses and veterinary technicians.

Veterinary medicine has made many important contributions to animal and human health. Included are dramatic reductions in animal sources of human exposure to tuberculosis and brucellosis. Safe and effective vaccines have been developed for prevention of many companion (pet) animal diseases—e.g., canine distemper and feline distemper (panleukopenia). The vaccine developed for control of Marek's disease in chickens was the first anticancer vaccine. Veterinarians developed surgical techniques, such as hip-joint replacement and organ transplants, that were later applied successfully to people.

A major challenge to veterinary medicine is adequately attending to the diversity of animal species. Veterinarians address the health needs of domestic animals, including cats, dogs, chickens, horses, cows, sheep, pigs, and goats; wildlife; zoo animals; pet birds; and ornamental fish. The sizes of animals that are treated vary from newborn hamsters to adult elephants, as do their economic values, which range from the undefinable value of pet animal companionship to the high monetary value of a winning racehorse. Medicating this variety of tame and wild animals requires special knowledge and skills.

On the basis of recognition by the World Health Organization (WHO) or the government of a country, there are about 450 veterinary degree programs worldwide. The level of veterinary training varies greatly among the various countries, and only about one-third of these programs designate the degree awarded as a doctor's degree. Professional training of veterinarians is commonly divided into two phases. The first, or basic science, phase consists of classroom study and laboratory work in the preclinical sciences, including the fields of anatomy, physiology, pathology, pharmacology, toxicology, nutrition, microbiology, and public health. The second phase focuses on the clinical sciences and includes classroom study of infectious and noninfectious diseases, diagnostic and clinical pathology, obstetrics, radiology, anesthesiology, surgery, and practice management and hands-on clinical experience in the college's veterinary teaching hospital. The clinical experience gives students the opportunity to treat sick animals, perform surgery, and communicate with animal owners. Student activities in the clinical setting are conducted under the supervision of graduate veterinarians on the faculty. Several important opportunities for additional training are available to graduate veterinarians. Internship (one-year) and residency (two-to-five-year) programs enable veterinarians to gain clinical proficiency in one or two medical specialties. Graduate veterinarians can also pursue advanced degree programs. Usually the field of advanced study is medically oriented, but some seek advanced degrees in areas such as business.

Most clinical-practice veterinarians treat only companion animals and usually within the practice's clinic, or animal hospital. A small proportion treat only food-producing animals or horses, most often by traveling to the location of the animal in a vehicle equipped for veterinary services in the field. Most of the remainder in clinical practice are in mixed practices, which deal with both small animals and large domestic animals such as cattle or horses. Some small-animal practices offer services for special species such as ornamental fish, caged birds, and reptiles. Some practices may limit work to a specific medical area such as surgery, dentistry, dermatology, or ophthalmology. Corporate-owned animal hospitals have increased in number and are often combined with a retail outlet for pet supplies.

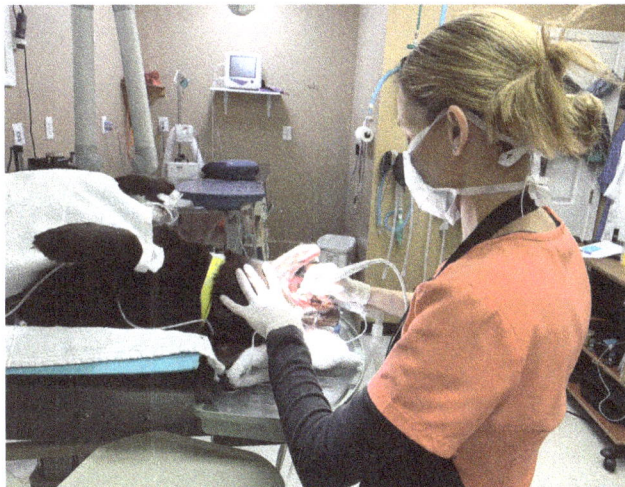

Veterinary medicine; small-animal dentistry: A veterinarian performs a dental procedure on a small dog

Veterinarians in academia administer the basic and clinical science programs of veterinary colleges. In addition, they conduct basic and clinical research, the latter of which may involve application of new instrumentation technologies for diagnosis and treatment of animal diseases. Included are echocardiography, laser lithotripsy, endoscopy, nuclear scintigraphy, ultrasonography, computed tomography (CT) scans, and magnetic resonance imaging.

Veterinary medicine intersects with private industry in such areas as marketing of animal-health products, monitoring of animal health in large commercial animal-production programs, and biomedical research. Veterinary specialists in industry work in the fields of toxicology, laboratory animal medicine, pathology, molecular biology, and genetic engineering. Pharmaceutical companies employ veterinarians in the development, safety testing, and clinical evaluation of drugs, chemicals, and biological products such as antibiotics and vaccines for animals and people.

National and local governments employ veterinarians in those agencies charged with public health, protection of the environment, agricultural research, food and drug safety, food-animal inspection, the health of imported animals, and the humane treatment of animals. Veterinarians working in public-health programs, for example, evaluate the safety of food-processing plants, restaurants, and water supplies. They also monitor and help control animal and human disease outbreaks. The increased threat of bioterrorism has given veterinarians vital roles in the protection of the food supply for animals and people and in early detection of use of zoonotic organisms as weapons. Veterinarians also work in aerospace; e.g., they have been scientific advisers on animal use in the U.S. space program and have been members of U.S. space shuttle crews. Veterinarians in military service perform biomedical research, care for military dogs, and protect troops through food-inspection and communicable-disease monitoring-and-control programs.

2

Animal Diseases and their Prevention

An animal disease can be defined as any impairment which hinders the normal functioning of an animal or its vital functions. Some of the diseases which can affect different animals are pseudorabies, equine viral arteritis, bird flu, rift valley fever and infectious bursal disease. This chapter has been carefully written to provide an easy understanding of these animal diseases as well as how they can be prevented.

Animal disease is an impairment of the normal state of an animal that interrupts or modifies its vital functions.

Concern with diseases that afflict animals dates from the earliest human contacts with animals and is reflected in early views of religion and magic. Diseases of animals remain a concern principally because of the economic losses they cause and the possible transmission of the causative agents to humans. The branch of medicine called veterinary medicine deals with the study, prevention, and treatment of diseases not only in domesticated animals but also in wild animals and in animals used in scientific research. The prevention, control, and eradication of diseases of economically important animals are agricultural concerns. Programs for the control of diseases communicable from animals to man, called zoonoses, especially those in pets and in wildlife, are closely related to human health. Further, the diseases of animals are of increasing importance, for a primary public-health problem throughout the world is animal-protein deficiency in the diet of humans. Indeed, both the United Nations Food and Agricultural Organization (FAO) and the World Health Organization (WHO) have been attempting to solve the problem of protein deficits in a world whose human population is rapidly expanding.

Importance

Economic Importance

About 50 percent of the world's population suffers from chronic malnutrition and hunger. Inadequate diet claims many thousands of lives each day. When the lack of adequate food to meet present needs for an estimated world population of more than 4,600,000,000 in the 1980s is coupled with the prediction that the population may increase to 7,000,000,000 by the year 2000, it becomes obvious that animal-food supplies must be increased. One way in which this might be accomplished is by learning to control the diseases that afflict animals throughout the world, especially in the developing nations of Asia and Africa, where the population is expanding most rapidly. Most of the information concerning animal diseases, however, applies to domesticated animals such as pigs, cattle, and sheep, which are relatively unimportant as food sources in these nations. Remarkably little is known of the diseases of the goat, the water buffalo, the camel, the elephant, the yak, the llama, or the alpaca; all are domesticated animals upon which the economies of many developing countries depend. It is in these countries that increased animal production resulting from the development of methods for the control and eradication of diseases affecting these animals is most urgently needed.

Despite the development of various effective methods of disease control, substantial quantities of meat and milk are lost each year throughout the world. In countries in which animal-disease control is not yet adequately developed, the loss of animal protein from disease is about 30 to 40 percent of the quantity available in certain underdeveloped areas. In addition, such countries also suffer losses resulting from poor husbandry practices.

Role in Human Disease

Animals have long been recognized as agents of human disease. Man has probably been bitten, stung, kicked, and gored by animals for as long as he has been on earth; in addition, early man sometimes became ill or died after eating the flesh of dead animals. In more recent times, man has discovered that many invertebrate animals are capable of transmitting causative agents of disease from man to man or from other vertebrates to man. Such animals, which act as hosts, agents, and carriers of disease, are important in causing and perpetuating human illness. Because about three-fourths of the important known zoonoses are associated with domesticated animals, including pets, the term zoonosis was originally defined as a group of diseases that man is able to acquire from domesticated animals. But this definition has been modified to include all human diseases (whether or not they manifest themselves in all hosts as apparent diseases) that are acquired from or transmitted to any other vertebrate animal. Thus, zoonoses are naturally occurring infections and infestations shared by man and other vertebrates.

Although the role of domesticated animals in many zoonoses is understood, the role of the numerous species of wild animals with which man is less intimately associated is not well understood. The discovery that diseases such as yellow fever, viral brain infections, plague, and numerous other important diseases involving man or his domesticated animals are fundamentally diseases of wildlife and exist independently of man and his civilization, however, has increased the significance of studying the nature of wildlife diseases.

Animals in Research: The Biomedical Model

Although in modern times the practice of veterinary medicine has been separated from that of human medicine, the observations of the physician and the veterinarian continue to add to the common body of medical knowledge. Of the more than 1,200,000 species of animals thus far identified, only a few have been utilized in research, even though it is likely that, for every known human disease, an identical or similar disease exists in at least one other animal species. Veterinary medicine plays an ever-increasing role in the health of man through the use of animals as biomedical models with similar disease counterparts in man. This use of animals as models is important because research on many genetic and chronic diseases of man cannot be carried out using humans.

Hundreds of thousands of mice and monkeys are utilized each year in research laboratories in the U.S. alone. Animal studies are used in the development of new surgical techniques (e.g., organ transplantations), in the testing of new drugs for safety, and in nutritional research. Animals are especially valuable in research involving chronic degenerative diseases, because such diseases can be induced in animals experimentally with relative ease. The importance of chronic degenerative diseases, such as cancer and cardiovascular diseases, has increased in parallel with the growing number of communicable diseases that have been brought under control.

Examples of animal diseases that are quite similar to commonly occurring human diseases include chronic emphysema in the horse; leukemia in cats and cattle; muscular dystrophies in chickens and mice; atherosclerosis in pigs and pigeons; blood-coagulation disorders and nephritis in dogs; gastric ulcers in swine; vascular aneurysms (permanent and abnormal blood-filled area of a blood vessel) in turkeys; diabetes mellitus in Chinese hamsters; milk allergy and gallstones in rabbits; hepatitis in dogs and horses; hydrocephalus (fluid in the head) and skin allergies in many species; epilepsy in dogs and gerbils; hereditary deafness in many small animals; cataracts in the eyes of dogs and mice; and urinary stones in dogs and cattle.

The study of animals with diseases similar to those that affect man has increased knowledge of the diseases in man; knowledge of nutrition, for example, based largely on the results of animal studies, has improved the health of animals, including man. Animal investigations have been used extensively in the treatment of shock, in open-heart surgery, in organ transplantations, and in the testing of new drugs. Other important contributions to human health undoubtedly will result from new research discoveries involving the study of animal diseases.

Role of Ecology

Epidemiology, the study of epidemics, is sometimes defined as the medical aspect of ecology, for it is the study of diseases in animal populations. Hence the epidemiologist is concerned with the interactions of organisms and their environments as related to the presence of disease. The multiple-causality concept of disease embraced by epidemiology involves combinations of environmental factors and host factors, in addition to the determination of the specific causative agent of a given disease. Environmental factors include geographical features, climate, and concentration of certain elements in soil and water. Host factors include age, breed, sex, and the physiological state of an animal as well as the general immunity of a herd resulting from previous contact with a disease. Epidemiology, therefore, is concerned with the determination of the individual animals that are affected by a disease, the environmental circumstances under which it may occur, the causative agents, and the ways in which transmission occurs in nature. The epidemiologist, who utilizes many scientific disciplines (e.g., medicine, zoology, mathematics, anthropology), attempts to determine the types of diseases that exist in a specific geographical area and to control them by modifying the environment.

Diseases in animal populations are characterized by certain features. Some outbreaks are termed sporadic diseases because they appear only occasionally in individuals within an animal population. Diseases normally present in an area are referred to as endemic, or enzootic, diseases, and they usually reflect a relatively stable relationship between the causative agent and the animals affected by it. Diseases that occasionally occur at higher than normal rates in animal populations are referred to as epidemic, or epizootic, diseases, and they generally represent an unstable relationship between the causative agent and affected animals.

The effect of diseases on a stable ecological system, which is the result of the dominance of some plants and animals and the subordination or extinction of others, depends on the degree to which the causative agents of diseases and their hosts are part of the system. Epidemic diseases result from an ecological imbalance; endemic diseases often represent a balanced state. Ecological imbalance and, hence, epidemic disease may be either naturally caused or induced by man. A breakdown in sanitation in a city, for example, offers conditions favourable for an increase in the rodent population, with the possibility that diseases such as plague may be introduced into and spread among the human population. In this case, an epidemic would result as much from an alteration in the environment as from the presence of the causative agent Pasteurella pestis, since, in relatively balanced ecological systems, the causative agent exists enzootically in the rodents (i.e., they serve as reservoirs for the disease) and seldom involves man. In a similar manner, an increase in the number of epidemics of viral encephalitis, a brain disease, in man has resulted from the ecological imbalance of mosquitoes and wild birds caused by man's exploitation of lowland for farming. Driven from their natural habitat of reeds and rushes, the wild birds, important natural hosts for the virus that causes the disease, are forced to feed near farms; mosquitoes transmit the virus from birds to cattle and man.

Detection and Diagnosis

Reactions of Tissue to Disease

As previously noted, disease may be defined as an injurious deviation from a normal physiological state of an organism sufficient to produce overt signs, or symptoms. The deviation may be either an obvious organic change in the tissue composing an organ or a functional disturbance whose organic changes are not obvious. The severity of the changes that occur in cells and tissues subjected to injurious agents is dependent upon both the sensitivity of the tissue concerned and the nature and time course of the agent. A mildly injurious agent that is present for short periods of time may either have little effect or stimulate cells to increased activity. Strongly injurious agents in prolonged contact with cells cause characteristic changes in them by interfering with normal cell processes. Most causative agents of disease fall into the latter category.

Characteristics of Cell and Tissue Changes

Changes in cells and tissues as a result of disease include degenerative and infiltrative changes. Degenerative changes are characterized by the deterioration of cells or a tissue from a higher to a lower form, especially to a less functionally active form. When chemical changes occur in the tissue, the process is one of degeneration. When the changes involve the accumulation of materials within the cells comprising tissues, the process is called infiltration. Diseases such as pneumonia, metal poisoning, or septicemia (the persistence of disease-causing bacteria in the bloodstream) may cause the mildest type of degeneration—parenchymatous changes, or cloudy swelling of the cells; the cells first affected are the specialized cells of the liver and the kidney. Serious cellular damage may cause the uptake of water by cells (hydropic degeneration), which lose their structural features as they fill with water. The causes for the accumulation in cells of abnormal amounts of fats (fatty infiltration and degeneration) have not yet been established with certainty but probably involve fat metabolism. Poisons such as phosphorus may cause sudden increases in the accumulation of fats in the liver. An abnormal protein material may accumulate in connective-tissue components of small arteries as a result of chronic pneumonia, chronic bacterial infections, and prolonged antitoxin production (in horses); the condition is known as amyloid degeneration and infiltration. Hyaline degeneration, characterized by tissues that become clear and appear glass-like, usually occurs in connective-tissue components of small blood vessels as a result of conditions that may occur in kidney structures (glomeruli) of animals with nephritis or in lymph glands of animals with tuberculosis. Certain structures (glomeruli) of animals with nephritis result in degeneration.

The condition in which mucus, a secretion of mucous membranes lining the inside surfaces of organs, is produced in excess and accumulates in greater than normal amounts is referred to as mucoid degeneration. Major causes of this condition include chronic irritation of mucous membranes and certain mucus-producing tumours. Abnormal amounts of glycogen, which is the principal storage carbohydrate of animals, may occur in the liver as a result of certain inherited diseases of animals; the condition is known as glycogen infiltration. The abnormal deposition of calcium salts, which is known as hypercalcification, may occur as a result of several diseases involving the blood vessels and the heart, the urinary system, the gallbladder, and the bonelike tissue called cartilage. Pigments (coloured molecules) from coal dust or asbestos dust may infiltrate the lungs of certain dogs in two types of lung disease: anthracosis and asbestosis. Abnormal amounts of iron-containing coloured molecules (hemosiderin) resulting from the breakdown of hemoglobin, the oxygen-carrying protein of red blood cells, are often deposited in the liver and the spleen after diseases that involve excessive breakdown of red blood cells. A dark-coloured molecule (melanin) occurs abnormally in the livers of certain sheep suffering from Dubin–Johnson syndrome and in certain tumours called melanomas. Uric acid infiltration, which occurs in poultry, is characterized by the deposition of uric acid salts.

Necrosis, the death of cells or tissues, takes place if the blood supply to tissues is restricted; poisons produced by microbes, chemical poisons, and extreme heat or electricity also may cause necrosis. The rotting of the dead tissue is known as gangrene.

Atrophy of animal tissue involves a process of tissue wasting, in which a decrease occurs in the size or number of functional cells—e.g., in inherited muscular dystrophy of chickens. Hypertrophy—an increase in the size of the cells in a tissue or an organ—occurs in heart muscle during diseases involving the heart valves, in certain pneumonias, and in some diseases of the endocrine glands. Aplasia is the term used when an entire organ is missing from an animal; hypoplasia indicates arrested or incomplete development of an organ, and hyperplasia an increase in the production of the number of cells—e.g., the persistent callus that forms on the elbows of some dogs. Metaplasia is used to describe the change of one cell type into another; it may occur in chronic irritation of tissues and in certain cancerous tumours.

Characteristics of Inflammatory Reactions

When tissues are injured, they become inflamed. The inflammation may be acute, in which case the inflammatory processes are active, or chronic, in which case the processes occur slowly and new connective tissue is formed. The reaction of inflamed tissues is a combination of defensive and repair mechanisms. Acute inflammation is characterized by redness, heat, swelling, sensitivity, and impaired function. Several types of acute inflammation are known. Mild acute inflammations of mucous membranes resulting in the production of thin watery material (exudate) are called catarrhal inflammations; parenchymatous inflammations occur in organs undergoing degeneration. If the exudate formed in response to an injury is of a serous nature—that is, resembling blood plasma—the process is called serous inflammation. In fibrinous inflammation, a protein (fibrin) forms on membranes, including those in the lungs. In suppurative inflammation, dead tissue is replaced with pus composed of colourless blood cells (leucocytes) and tissue juices.

During the inflammatory reaction, the injured tissue is surrounded by an area of rapidly dividing cells. Specialized cells called macrophages enter the tissue and remove blood and tissue debris. Other cells, called neutrophils, ingest disease-causing bacteria and other foreign material. In chronic inflammations, the connective tissue contains fibroblasts, cells that divide and form new connective, or scar, tissue.

Characteristics of Circulatory Disturbances

An increase in the rate of blood flow to a body part, which is referred to by the term congestion, or hyperemia, occurs during inflammation; a diminished blood flow to tissues is referred to by the term ischemia, or a local anemia. Examples of hemorrhage, the escape of blood from vessels, include epistaxis, or nosebleeds, in racehorses; hematemesis, or regurgitation of blood, in dogs with uremia; hemoptysis, or blood loss from lungs; hematuria, or blood in urine, of cattle with inflammation of the urinary bladder. Edema, a condition that is characterized by abnormal accumulations of fluid in tissues, occurs not only in a tissue during inflammation but also over the entire body if the concentration of blood-serum proteins, especially albumin, is low. A thrombosis, which is a blood clot in a blood vessel, may block or slow circulation of blood to tissues; if blood vessels become blocked, the condition is known as an embolism. The term infarction describes the necrosis that occurs in tissues whose blood supply is blocked by an embolism.

Methods of Examination

Before an unhealthy animal receives treatment, an attempt is made to diagnose the disease. Both clinical findings, which include symptoms that are obvious to a nonspecialist and clinical signs that can be appreciated only by a veterinarian, and laboratory test results may be necessary to establish the cause of a disease. A clinical examination should indicate if the animal is in good physical condition, is eating adequately, is bright and alert, and is functioning in an apparently normal manner. Many disease processes are either inflammatory or result from tumours. Malignant tumours (e.g., melanomas in horses, squamous cell carcinomas in small animals) tend to spread rapidly and usually cause death. Other diseases cause the circulatory disturbances or the degenerative and infiltrative changes that are summarized in the preceding topic. If a specific diagnosis is not possible, the symptoms of the animal are treated.

A case record of the information pertaining to an animal (or to a herd of animals) that is suspected of having a disease is begun at the time the animal is taken to a veterinarian (or the veterinarian visits the animal) and is continued through treatment. It includes a description of the animal (age, species, sex, breed); the owner's report; the animal's history; a description of the preliminary examination; clinical findings resulting from an examination of body systems; results of specific laboratory tests; diagnosis regarding a specific cause for the disease (etiology); outlook (prognosis); treatment; case progress; termination; autopsy, if performed; and the utilization of scientific references, if applicable.

The veterinarian must diagnose a disease on the basis of a variety of examinations and tests, since he obviously cannot interrogate the animal. Methods used in the preparation of a diagnosis include inspection—a visual examination of the animal; palpation—the application of firm pressure with the fingers to tissues to determine characteristics such as abnormal shapes and possible tumours, the presence of pain, and tissue consistency; percussion—the application of a short, sharp blow to a tissue to provoke an audible response from body parts directly beneath; auscultation—the act of listening to sounds that are produced by the body during the performance of functions (e.g., breathing, intestinal movements); smells—the recognition of characteristic odours associated with certain diseases; and miscellaneous diagnostic procedures, such as eye examinations, the collection of urine, and heart, esophageal, and stomach studies.

Deviation of various characteristics from the normal, observation of which constitutes the general inspection of an animal, is a useful aid in diagnosing disease. The general inspection includes examination of appearance; behaviour; body condition; respiratory movements; state of skin, coat, and abdomen; and various common actions.

The appearance of an animal may be of diagnostic significance; small size in a pig may result from retardation of growth, which is caused by hog-cholera virus. Observation of the behaviour of an animal is of value in diagnosing neurological diseases; e.g., muscle spasms occur in lockjaw (tetanus) in dogs, nervousness and convulsions in dogs with distemper, dullness in horses with equine viral encephalitis, and excitement in animals suffering from lead poisoning. Subtle behavioral changes may not be noticeable. The general condition of the body is of value in diagnosing diseases that cause excessive leanness (emaciation), including certain cancers, or other chronic diseases, such as a deficiency in the output of the adrenal glands or tuberculosis. Defective teeth also may point to malnutrition and result in emaciation.

The respiratory movements of an animal are important diagnostic criteria; breathing is rapid in young animals, in small animals, and in animals whose body temperature is higher than normal. Specific respiratory movements are characteristic of certain diseases—e.g., certain movements in horses with heaves (emphysema) or the abdominal breathing of animals suffering from painful lung diseases. The appearance of the skin and hair may indicate dehydration by lack of pliability and lustre; or the presence of parasites such as lice, mites, or fleas; or the presence of ringworm infections and allergic reactions by the skin changes they cause. The poisoning of sheep by molybdenum in their hay may be diagnosed by the loss of colour in the wool of black sheep. Distension of the abdomen may indicate bloat in cattle or colic in horses.

Abnormal activities may have special diagnostic meaning to the veterinarian. Straining during urination is associated with bladder stones; increased frequency of urination is associated with kidney disease (nephritis), bladder infections, and a disease of the pituitary gland (diabetes insipidus). Excessive salivation and grinding of teeth may be caused by an abnormality in the mouth. Coughing is associated with pneumonia. Some diseases cause postural changes: for example, a horse with tetanus may stand in a stiff manner. An abnormal gait in an animal made to move may furnish evidence as to the cause of a disease, as louping ill in sheep.

Clinical Examination

Following the general inspection of an animal thought to have contracted a disease, a more thorough clinical examination is necessary, during which various features of the animal are studied. These include the visible mucous membranes (conjunctiva of the eye, nasal mucosa, inside surface of the mouth, and tongue); the eye itself; and such body surfaces as the ears, horns (if present), and limbs. In addition, the pulse rate and the temperature are measured.

The veterinarian examines the visible mucous membranes of the eye, nose, and mouth to determine if jaundice, hemorrhages, or anemia are present. The conjunctiva, or lining of the eye, may exhibit pus in pinkeye infections, have a yellow appearance in jaundice, or exhibit small hemorrhages in certain systemic diseases. Examination of the nose may reveal ulcers and vesicles (small sacs containing liquid), as in foot-and-mouth disease, a viral disease of cattle, or vesicular exanthema, a viral disease of swine. Ulceration of the tongue may be apparent in animals suffering from actinobacillosis, a disease of bacterial origin.

A detailed examination of the eye may show abnormalities of the cornea resulting from such diseases as infectious hepatitis in dogs, bovine catarrhal fever, and equine influenza. Cataract, a condition in which the passage of light through the lens of the eye is obstructed, may result from a disorder of carbohydrate metabolism (diabetes mellitus), infections, or a hereditary defect.

An elevated temperature, or fever, resulting from the multiplication of disease-causing organisms may be the earliest sign of disease. The increase in temperature activates the body mechanisms that are necessary to fight off foreign substances. Measuring the pulse rate is useful in determining the character of the heartbeat and of the circulatory system.

Tests as Diagnostic Aids

In many cases, the final diagnosis of an animal disease is dependent upon a laboratory test. Some involve measuring the amount of certain chemical constituents of the blood or body fluids, determining the presence of toxins (poisons), or examining the urine and feces. Other tests are designed to identify the causative agents of the disease. The removal and examination of tissue or other material from the body (biopsy) is used to diagnose the nature of abnormalities such as tumours. Specific skin tests are used to confirm the diagnoses of various diseases—e.g., tuberculosis and Johne's disease in cattle and glanders in horses.

Confirmation of the presence in the blood of abnormal quantities of certain constituents aids in diagnosing certain diseases. Abnormal levels of protein in the blood are associated with some cancers of the bone, such as multiple myeloma in horses and dogs. Animals with diabetes mellitus have a high level of the carbohydrate glucose and the steroid cholesterol in the blood. The combination of an increase in the blood level of cholesterol and a decrease in the level of iodine bound to protein indicates hypothyroidism (underactive thyroid gland). A low level of calcium in the serum component of blood confirms milk fever in lactating dairy cattle. An increase in the activities of certain enzymes (biological catalysts) in the blood indicates liver damage. An increase in the blood level of the bile constituent bilirubin is used as a diagnostic test for hemolytic crisis, a disease in which red blood cells are rapidly destroyed by organisms such as Babesia species in dogs and in cattle and Anaplasma species in cattle.

The examination of the formed elements of blood, including the oxygen-carrying red blood cells (erythrocytes), the white blood cells (neutrophils, eosinophils, basophils, lymphocytes, and monocytes), and the platelets, which function in blood coagulation, is helpful in diagnosing certain diseases. Examination of the blood cells of cattle may reveal abnormal lymphocytic cells characteristic of leukemia. Low numbers of leucocytes indicate the presence of viral diseases, such as hog cholera and infectious hepatitis in dogs. Neutrophil levels increase in chronic bacterial diseases, such as canine pneumonia and uterine infections in female animals. Elevated monocyte levels occur in chronic granulomatous diseases; e.g., histoplasmosis and tuberculosis. Canine parasitism and allergic skin disorders are characterized by elevated eosinophil levels. Prolonged clotting time may be associated with a deficiency of platelets.

Anemia has many causes. They include hemorrhages from blood loss after injuries; the destruction of red blood cells by the rickettsia Haemobartonella felis in cats; incompatible blood transfusions in dogs; the inadequate production of normal red blood cells, which occurs in iron or cobalt deficiency after exposure to radioactive substances; general malnutrition; and contact with substances that depress the activity of bone marrow.

Poisonings occur commonly in animals. Some species are more sensitive to certain poisons than others. Swine develop mercury poisoning if they eat too much grain that has been treated with mercury compounds to retard spoilage. Dogs may be poisoned by the arsenic found in pesticides or by strychnine, which is found in rat poison. Many plants are poisonous if eaten, such as bracken fern, which poisons cattle and horses, and ragwort, which contains a substance poisonous to the liver of cattle.

Examination of an animal's urine may reveal evidence of kidney diseases or diseases of the entire urinary system or a generalized systemic disease. The presence of protein in the urine of dogs indicates acute kidney disease (nephritis). Although constituents of bile normally are found in the urine of dogs, the quantity increases in dogs with the presence of infectious hepatitis, a disease of the liver. The presence of abnormal amounts of the simple carbohydrate glucose and of ketone bodies (organic compounds involved in metabolism) in an animal's urine is used to diagnose diabetes mellitus, a disease in which the pancreas cannot form adequate quantities of a substance (insulin) important in regulating carbohydrate metabolism. The urine of horses with azoturia (excessive quantities of nitrogen-containing compounds in the urine) or muscle breakdown may contain a dark-coloured molecule called myoglobin.

The presence of eggs or parts of worms in the excrement of animals suspected of suffering from intestinal parasites, such as roundworms, tapeworms, or flatworms, aids in diagnosis. Feces that are light in colour, have a rancid odour, contain fat, and are poorly formed may indicate the existence of a chronic disease of the pancreas. Clay-coloured fatty feces suggest obstruction of the bile duct, which conveys bile to the intestine during digestion.

The identification of a disease-causing microorganism within an animal enables the veterinarian to choose the best drug for therapy. Agglutination tests, which utilize serum samples of animals and microorganisms suspected of causing a disease, many times confirm the presence of the following bacterial diseases: brucellosis in cattle and swine, salmonellosis in swine, leptospirosis in cattle, and actinobacillosis in swine and cattle. Other tests measure the antibodies (specific proteins formed in response to a foreign substance in the body) formed against a disease-causing agent, such as those that cause brucellosis, foot-and-mouth disease, infectious hepatitis in dogs, and fowl pest.

The modern veterinary diagnostic laboratory performs, in addition to the tests mentioned, tests of cells in the bone marrow; specific-organ-function tests (liver, kidney, pancreas, thyroid, adrenal, and pituitary glands); radioisotope tests, tissue biopsies, and histochemical analyses; and tests concerning blood coagulation and body fluids.

Infectious and Noninfectious Diseases

Diseases may be either infectious or noninfectious. The term infection, as observed earlier, implies an interaction between two living organisms, called the host and the parasite. Infection is a type of parasitism, which may be defined as the state of existence of one organism (the parasite) at the expense of another (the host). Agents (e.g., certain viruses, bacteria, fungi, protozoans, worms, and arthropods) capable of producing disease are pathogens. The term pathogenicity refers to the ability of a parasite to enter a host and produce disease; the degree of pathogenicity—that is, the ability of an organism to cause infection—is known as virulence. The capacity of a virulent organism to cause infection is influenced both by the characteristics of the organism and by the ability of the host to repel the invasion and to prevent injury. A pathogen may be virulent for one host but not for another. Pneumococcal bacteria, for example, have a low virulence for mice and are not found in them in nature; if introduced experimentally into a mouse, however, the bacteria overwhelm its body defenses and cause death.

Many pathogens (e.g., the bacterium that causes anthrax) are able to live outside the animal's body until conditions occur that are favourable for entering and infecting it. Pathogens enter the body in various ways—by penetrating the skin or an eye, by being eaten with food, or by being breathed into the lungs. After their entry into a host, pathogens actively multiply and produce disease by interfering with the functions of specific organs or tissues of the host.

Before a disease becomes established in a host, the barrier known as immunity must be overcome. Defense against infection is provided by a number of chemical and mechanical barriers, such as the skin, mucous membranes and secretions, and components of the blood and other body fluids. Antibodies, which are proteins formed in response to a specific substance (called an antigen) recognized by the body as foreign, are another important factor in preventing infection. Immunity among animals varies with species, general health, heredity, environment, and previous contact with a specific pathogen.

As certain bacterial species multiply, they may produce and liberate poisons, called exotoxins, into the tissues; other bacterial pathogens contain toxins, called endotoxins, which produce disease only when liberated at the time of death of the bacterial cell. Some bacteria, such as certain species of Clostridium and Bacillus, have inactive forms called spores, which may remain viable (i.e., capable of developing into active organisms) for many years; spores are highly resistant to environmental conditions such as heat, cold, and chemical compounds called disinfectants, which are able to kill many active bacteria.

The term infestation indicates that animals, including spiny-headed worms (Acanthocephala), roundworms (Nematoda), flatworms (Platyhelminthes), and arthropods such as lice, fleas, mites, and ticks, are present in or on the body of a host. An infestation is not necessarily parasitic.

Noninfectious diseases are not caused by virulent pathogens and are not communicable from one animal to another. They may be caused by hereditary factors or by the environment in which an animal lives. Many metabolic diseases are caused by an unsuitable alteration, sometimes brought about by man, in an animal's genetic constitution or in its environment. Metabolic diseases usually result from a disturbance in the normal balance of the physiological mechanisms that maintain stability, or homeostasis. Examples of metabolic diseases include overproduction or underproduction of hormones, which control specific body processes; nutritional deficiencies; poisoning from such agents as insecticides, fungicides, herbicides, fluorine, and poisonous plants; and inherited deficiencies in the ability to synthesize active forms of specific enzymes, which are the proteins that control the rates of chemical reactions in the body.

Excessive inbreeding (i.e., the mating of related animals) among all domesticated animal species has resulted in an increase in the number of metabolic diseases and an increase in the susceptibility of certain animals to infectious diseases.

Zoonoses

As stated previously, zoonoses are human diseases acquired from or transmitted to any other vertebrate animal. Zoonotic diseases are common in currently developing countries throughout the world and constitute, with starvation, the major threat to human health. More than 150 such diseases are known.

Zoonoses may be separated into four principal types, depending on the mechanisms of transmission and epidemiology. One type includes the direct zoonoses, such as rabies and brucellosis, which are maintained in nature by one vertebrate species. The transmission cycle of the cyclozoonoses, of which tapeworm infections are an example, requires at least two different vertebrate species. Both vertebrate and invertebrate animals are required as intermediate hosts in the transmission to humans of metazoonoses; arboviral and trypanosomal diseases are good examples of metazoonoses. The cycles of saprozoonoses (for example, histoplasmosis) may require, in addition to vertebrate hosts, specific environmental locations or reservoirs.

Most animals that serve as reservoirs for zoonoses are domesticated and wild animals with which man commonly associates. People in occupations such as veterinary medicine and public health, therefore, have a greater exposure to zoonoses than do those in occupations less closely concerned with animals.

In addition to the numerous human diseases spread by contact with the parasitic worm helminth and by contact with arthropods, many diseases are transmitted by the bites and venom of certain animals; poisonous or diseased food animals also transmit diseases. Dog bites may seriously injure tissues and also can transmit bacterial infections and rabies, a disease of viral origin. The bite of a diseased rat may transmit any of several diseases to man, including plague, salmonellosis, leptospirosis, and rat-bite fevers. Cat scratch disease may be transmitted through cat bites, and the deadly herpes B virus can spread by monkey bites. The bites of venomous snakes and fish account for considerable human discomfort and death. About 200 of the 2,500 known species of snakes can cause human disease. One estimate for snakebite deaths worldwide is 30,000 to 40,000 per year, the vast majority of them in Asia. Poisonous wild animals inadvertently used for food include animals harbouring the anthrax bacillus and those containing the causative agents of salmonellosis, trichinosis, and fish-tapeworm infection. The flesh of various types of fish is toxic to man. Japanese puffers, for example, contain the poisonous chemical compound tetrodotoxin; scombroid fish harbour Proteus morganii, which causes gastrointestinal diseases; and mullet and surmullet can cause nervous disturbances.

Approaches to the control of zoonoses differ according to the type under consideration. Because the majority of direct zoonoses and cyclozoonoses and some saprozoonoses are most effectively controlled by techniques involving the animal host, methods used to combat these diseases are almost entirely the responsibility of veterinary medicine. A good example is the elimination of stray dogs, for they are an important factor in the control of zoonoses such as rabies, hydatid disease, and visceral larva migrans. In addition, the control of diseases such as brucellosis and tuberculosis in cattle involves a combination of methods—mass immunization, diagnosis, slaughter of infected animals, environmental disinfection, and quarantine. Several supportive measures for the control of disease are useful in some cases. Air-sanitation measures are helpful in direct zoonoses in which human illness is spread by droplets or dust, and zoonotic infections that are spread through a fluid medium, such as water or milk, sometimes can be controlled. Heat, cold, and irradiation are effective in killing the immature forms of Trichinella spiralis, the causative agent of trichinosis, in meat; and certain antibiotic drugs help to prevent deterioration of food.

The control of metazoonoses may be directed at the infected vertebrate hosts, at the infected invertebrate host, or at both. Particularly effective in this instance has been the use of chemical insecticides to attack the invertebrate carriers of specific infections, even though several difficulties have been encountered—for example, the inaccessibility of the invertebrate to the chemicals, which occurs with organisms that breed in swiftly flowing waters or in dense vegetation, and the development of insecticide resistance by the organisms. Insecticides are used to destroy the mosquitoes that spread malaria (Anopheles). Mechanical filters placed across irrigation ditches help to prevent the dissemination of the snails that transmit Schistosoma mansoni, a parasitic flatworm.

Disease Prevention, Control and Eradication

Prevention is the first line of defense against disease. At least four preventive techniques are available for use in the prevention of disease in an animal population. One is the exclusion of causative agents of disease from specific geographic areas, or quarantine. A second preventive tool utilizes control methods such as immunization, environmental control, and chemical agents to protect specific animal populations from endemic diseases, diseases normally present in an area. The third preventive measure concerns the mass education of people about disease prevention. Finally, early diagnosis of illness among members of an animal population is important so that disease manifestations do not become too severe and so that affected animals can be more easily managed and treated.

Quarantine—the restriction of movement of animals suffering from or exposed to infections such as bluetongue and scrapie (in sheep), foot-and-mouth disease (in cattle), and rabies (in dogs)—is one of the oldest tools of preventive medicine. It was applied to domesticated animals as early as Roman times. The establishment of international livestock quarantine in the United States in 1890 provided for the holding of all imported cattle, sheep, and swine at the port of entry for 90, 15, and 15 days, respectively. In this way, such diseases as Nairobi sheep disease, surra, and infections caused by Brucella melitensis were eliminated or excluded from the United States, but international quarantine barriers did not prevent the entry of bluetongue, scrapie, and the tick Rhipicephalus evertsi, which is a carrier for several animal diseases. On the other hand, long-term quarantine of all dogs entering Great Britain has been effective since its initiation in 1919 (the quarantine also includes cats). It is possible that aircraft may pose new problems regarding livestock-disease quarantine since many disease carriers (e.g., insects and viruses) may be accidentally brought by plane into a country.

Mass immunization as a preventive technique has the advantage of allowing the resistant animal freedom of movement, unlike environmental control, in which the animal is confined to the controlled area; immunization may, however, provide only short-lived and partial protection. Mass-inoculation techniques against diseases such as Newcastle disease in chickens and distemper in mink and dogs have been successful. Animal diseases have been prevented by methods involving environmental control, including the maintenance of safe water supplies, the hygienic disposal of animal excrement, air sanitation, pest control, and the improvement of animal housing. One specific environmental program, called the portable-calf-pen system, involves routine movement of the pens to avoid a concentration of specific pathogens in them. Other programs involve the utilization of automatic and sanitary watering and feeding equipment and buildings with environmental controls. The use of chemical compounds to prevent illness (chemoprophylaxis) includes a variety of pesticides, which are used to kill insects that transmit diseases, and substances either used internally or applied to the animal's body to prevent the transmission or the development of a disease. An example is the use of sulfonamide drugs in the drinking water of poultry to prevent coccidiosis. Environmental-control methods in the poultry industry have resulted in the most efficient means of poultry production developed thus far.

The early detection of a disease in a population of animals—a herd of cattle, for example—is particularly useful in controlling certain chronic infectious diseases, such as mastitis, brucellosis, and tuberculosis, as well as certain noninfectious diseases such as bloat. Laboratory tests—the agglutination test in pullorum disease, the tuberculin skin test for tuberculosis, the examination of feces for eggs of specific parasites, the physical and chemical tests performed on milk to diagnose bovine mastitis—are used for the early detection of diseases in an animal population.

Methods of disease control and eradication have been successful in various countries. In the United States, for example, the test-and-slaughter technique, in which simple tests are used to confirm the existence of diseased animals that are then slaughtered, has been of great value in controlling infectious and hereditary diseases, including dourine, a venereal disease in horses, fowl plague, and foot-and-mouth disease in cattle and deer. Bovine tuberculosis has been eliminated from Denmark, Finland, and The Netherlands and reduced to a low level in various other countries, including Great Britain, Japan, the United States, and Canada, by the test-and-slaughter method. Many infectious diseases have been eradicated from Great Britain—sheep pox, rinderpest, pleuropneumonia, glanders, and rabies. Diseases eliminated from Australia by a combination of methods—control of agents that carry disease, the test-and-slaughter technique, the use of chemical agents, and, more recently, biological control—include hog cholera, rinderpest, scrapie, glanders, surra, rabies, and foot-and-mouth disease.

In biological control, enemies of the agents that transmit the disease, enemies of the reservoir host, or a specific parasite are introduced into the environment. If a natural enemy of the tsetse fly could be found, for example, African sleeping sickness in man and trypanosomiasis in cattle could be controlled in West Africa. Successful biological control of the European-rabbit population in

Australia has been accomplished through the use of the myxomatosis virus, which is transmitted by mosquitoes and causes the formation of malignant tumours. Although the Brazilian white rabbit is relatively unaffected by the virus, it causes rapid death in the European rabbit. The elimination of the European rabbit in France by the virus was accompanied by a decrease in tick-borne typhus in people, suggesting that the rabbit may be a significant intermediate host for the causative agent, Rickettsia conorii. Screwworms, an immature form of the fly Cochliomyia hominivorax, have been eradicated in the United States by the release of more than 3,000,000,000 sterilized males.

Disease control and elimination programs require many sophisticated techniques in addition to diagnosis and the slaughter of affected animals. They include: the control of insects known to transmit diseases; the cooperation of animal owners; the development through research of new diagnostic tests for use on large populations; the eradication of animal species from areas in which they are known to transmit disease; sterilization of strains of animals known to carry inheritable metabolic diseases; and effective meat inspection.

Pseudorabies

Aujeszky's disease, usually called pseudorabies in the United States, is a viral disease in swine that has been endemic in most parts of the world. It is caused by *Suid herpesvirus 1* (SuHV-1). Aujeszky's disease is considered to be the most economically important viral disease of swine in areas where classical swine fever (hog cholera) has been eradicated. Other mammals, such as cattle, sheep, goats, cats, dogs, and raccoons, are also susceptible. The disease is usually fatal in these animal species.

The term "pseudorabies" is found inappropriate by many people, as SuHV-1 is a herpesvirus and has a DNA based genome (rabies virus has an RNA based genome).

Research on SuHV-1 in pigs has pioneered animal disease control with genetically modified vaccines. SuHV-1 is now used in model studies of basic processes during lytic herpesvirus infection, and for unravelling molecular mechanisms of herpesvirus neurotropism.

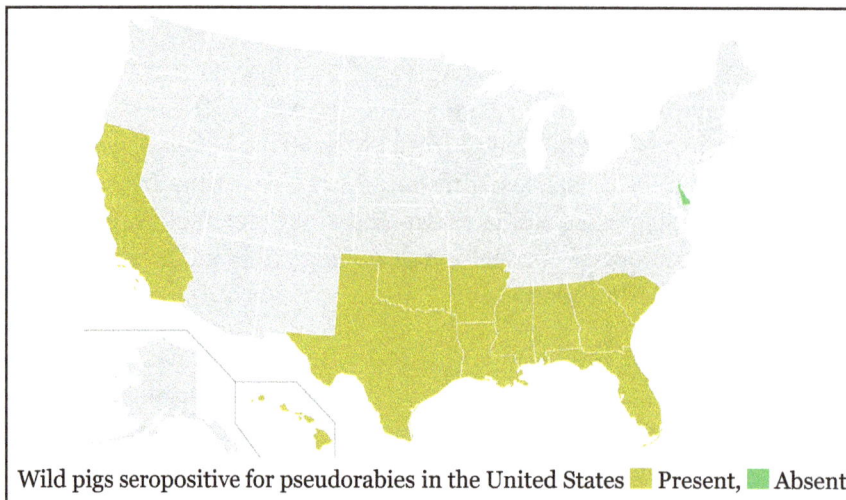

Wild pigs seropositive for pseudorabies in the United States ▪ Present, ▪ Absent

In 1902, a Hungarian veterinarian, Aladár Aujeszky, demonstrated a new infectious agent in a dog, ox, and cat, and showed it caused the same disease in swine and rabbits. In the following decades the infection was found in several European countries, especially in cattle, where local intense pruritus (itching) is a characteristic symptom. And in the United States a well known disease in cattle called "mad itch" was concluded to be in fact Aujeszky's disease.

The virus is shed in the saliva and nasal secretions of swine infected by the respiratory route. Aerosolization of the virus and transmission by fomites also may occur. The virus may potentially survive for seven hours in humid air, and it may survive on well water for up to seven hours, in green grass, soil, and feces for up to two days, in contaminated feed for up to three days, and in straw bedding for up to four days.

Diagnosis is made mainly by virus isolation in tissue cultures, or through ELISA or PCR tests. Vaccines are available for swine. The infection has been eradicated in a number of European countries. In the United States, the domestic swine population in 2004 was declared free of Aujeszky's disease, though the infection still remains in feral pig populations.

Clinical Signs

Respiratory infection is usually asymptomatic in pigs more than 2 months old, but it can cause abortion, high mortality in piglets, and coughing, sneezing, fever, constipation, depression, seizures, ataxia, circling, and excess salivation in piglets and mature pigs. Mortality in piglets less than one month of age is close to 100%, but it is less than 10% in pigs between one and six months of age. Pregnant swine can reabsorb their litters or deliver mummified, stillborn, or weakened piglets. In cattle, symptoms include intense itching followed by neurological signs and death. In dogs, symptoms include intense itching, jaw and pharyngeal paralysis, howling, and death Any infected secondary host generally only lives two to three days.

Genital infection appears to have been common in a great part of the 20th century in many European countries in swine herds, where boars from boar centres were used for natural service of sows or gilts. This disease manifestation has always been asymptomatic in affected pigs, and presence of the infection on a farm was detected only because of cases in cattle showing pruritus on the hindquarters.

In susceptible animals other than swine, infection is usually fatal, and the affected animals most often show intense pruritus in a skin area. Pruritus in Aujeszky's disease is considered a phantom sensation as virus has never been found at the site of pruritus.

Pathogenicity and Virulence of SuHV-1

The epidemiology of Aujeszky's disease varies with the pathogenicity or virulence of the virus strain involved. This is best illustrated by the development of the severity of the disease in Denmark, where import of swine had been forbidden for decades up to 1972. Before 1964 only genital strains were spread, but then respiratory strains appeared, which subsequently were spread rapidly over the country, mainly by the trade of animals. In the late 1970's more virulent strains developed. The disease in swine became much more severe, outbreaks of respiratory disease in cattle rose dramatically, and the infection was spread airborne to other swine herds. The higher virulence of these virus strains was associated with a certain ability to create syncytia (cell fusion) in tissue cultures (syncytial virus strains). Comprehensive restriction fragment pattern analyses of virus DNA have documented that the more virulent strains had not been introduced from abroad but had developed in two steps from the original Danish strains. The correlation between high virulence of virus strains and syncytium formation in tissue cultures was confirmed by examinations of isolates from other countries. This second step in the severity development of the disease in Denmark caused the decision to eradicate. New outbreaks after the eradication of the indigenous infection by the end of 1985 were all caused by foreign highly virulent, syncytial strains introduced by airborne transmission from Germany.

Briefly, SuHV-1 is spread either genitally or respiratorily. Genital strains have been found to be non-syncytial. Respiratory strains may be of relatively low or of high virulence. In Europe, syncytial strains have been found to be highly virulent.

Epidemiology

Populations of wild boar, or feral hogs (*Sus scrofa*), in the US commonly contract and spread the virus throughout their range. Mortality is highest in young piglets. Pregnant sows often abort when infected. Otherwise healthy male adults (boars) are typically latent carriers, that is, they harbor and transmit the virus without displaying signs or suffering disability.

Swine (both domestic and feral) are usual reservoirs for this virus, though it does affect other species. Aujeszky's disease has been reported in other mammals, including brown bears, and black bears, Florida panthers, raccoons, coyotes, and whitetail deer. In most cases, contact with pigs or pig products was either known or suspected. Outbreaks in farm fur species in Europe (mink and foxes) have been associated with feeding contaminated pig products. Many other species can be experimentally infected. Humans are not potential hosts.

Cattle have been found to be infected either by the respiratory or the vaginal route (iatrogenic cases disregarded). Primary infection of mucous membranes of the upper respiratory tract is associated with head pruritus, while lung infection results in chest pruritus. Vaginal infection of bovines, which regularly show pruritus of the hindquarters, has been found to be associated with a concurrent genital infection in swine on the same premises, and investigations have evidenced that the vaginal infection of cattle had been sexually transmitted by man from infected sows (zoophilia/bestiality). Genital infection in swine herds has been closely correlated with the use of boars from boar centres for natural service of sows.

Transmission

Aujeszky's disease is highly contagious. The infection is commonly considered to be transmitted among swine through nose-to-nose contact, because the virus is mostly present in nasal and oral areas. This notion, however, is contradicted by results from epidemiological studies, according to which the decisive spread within herds occurs by air currents over many meters. Correspondingly, the risk of airborne transmission of highly virulent virus strains from acutely infected herds to other swine herds has been found to be very high. The infection has been found transmitted over distances of many kilometers. Otherwise, the infection is most often transmitted into herds by introduction of acutely or latently infected pigs.

Prevention

Although no specific treatment for acute infection with SuHV-1 is available, vaccination can alleviate clinical signs in pigs of certain ages. Typically, mass vaccination of all pigs on the farm with a modified live virus vaccine is recommended. Intranasal vaccination of sows and neonatal piglets one to seven days old, followed by intramuscular (IM) vaccination of all other swine on the premises, helps reduce viral shedding and improve survival. The modified live virus replicates at the site of injection and in regional lymph nodes. Vaccine virus is shed in such low levels, mucous transmission to other animals is minimal. In gene-deleted vaccines, the thymidine kinase gene has also been deleted; thus, the virus cannot infect and replicate in neurons. Breeding herds are recommended to be vaccinated quarterly, and finisher pigs should be vaccinated after levels of maternal antibody decrease. Regular vaccination results in excellent control of the disease. Concurrent antibiotic therapy via feed and IM injection is recommended for controlling secondary bacterial pathogens.

Equine Viral Arteritis

Equine viral arteritis (EVA) is a disease of horses caused by *Alphaarterivirus equid*, an RNA virus. It is the only species in the genus *Alphaarterivirus*, and that is the only genus in the *Equarterivirinae* subfamily. The virus which causes EVA was first isolated in 1953, but the disease has afflicted equine animals worldwide for centuries. It has been more common in some breeds of horses in the United States, but there is no breed "immunity". In the UK, it is a notifiable disease. There is no known human hazard.

Signs and Symptoms

The signs shown depend on the horse's age, the strain of the infecting virus, the condition of the horse and the route by which it was infected. Most horses with EVA infection don't show any signs; if a horse does show symptoms, these can vary greatly in severity. Following infection, the first sign is fever, peaking at 41 °C (106 °F), followed by various signs such as depression, nasal discharge, "pink eye" (conjunctivitis), swelling over the eye (supraorbital edema), urticaria, and swelling of the limbs and under the belly (the ventral abdomen) which may extend to the udder in mares or the scrotum of male horses. More unusual signs include abortion in pregnant mares, and, most likely in foals, severe respiratory distress and death.

Cause

EVA is caused by an arterivirus called equine arteritis virus (EAV). Arteriviruses are small, enveloped, animal viruses with an icosahedral core containing a positive-sense RNA genome. As well as equine arteritis virus the Arterivirus family includes porcine reproductive and respiratory syndrome virus (PRRSV), lactate dehydrogenase elevating virus (LDV) of mice and simian haemorrhagic fever virus (SHFV).

There are a number of routes of transmission of the virus. The most frequent is the respiratory route. The virus can also be spread by the venereal route, including by artificial insemination. Stallions may become carriers.

Diagnosis

Because of the variability of symptoms, diagnosis is by laboratory testing. Blood samples, nasal swabs and semen can be used for isolation of the virus, detection of the viral RNA by polymerase chain reaction (PCR), and detection of antibodies by ELISA and virus neutralisation tests.

Prevention

A vaccine is available in the UK and Europe, however in laboratory tests it is not possible to distinguish between antibodies produced as a result of vaccination and those produced in response to infection with the virus. Management also plays an important part in the prevention of EVA.

Duck Plague

Duck plague (also known as duck viral enteritis) is a worldwide disease caused by Anatid alpha-herpesvirus 1 (AnHV-1) of the family *Herpesviridae* that causes acute disease with high mortality rates in flocks of ducks, geese, and swans. It is spread both vertically and horizontally—through contaminated water and direct contact. Migratory waterfowl are a major factor in the spread of this disease as they are often asymptomatic carriers of disease. The incubation period is three to seven days. Birds as young as one week old can be infected. DEV is not zoonotic.

Clinical Signs and Diagnosis

Upon exposure to DEV there is a 3-7 day for domestic fowl and up to a 14 day for wildfowl incubation period for the onset of symptoms. Sudden and persistent increases in flock mortality is often the first observation of DEV. Symptoms in individual birds include loss of appetite, decreased egg production (nearing 20-40% decreases), nasal discharge, increased thirst, diarrhea, ataxia, tremors, a drooped-wing appearance, and in males a prolapsed penis. Mortality rates for DEV may reach 90 percent. Death usually occurs within 5 days after onset of symptoms. The clinical signs of DEV "vary with virulence of virus strain, species, sex, and immune system status" of the host.

Due to the formation of diphtheroid plaques on the eyelids and the mucosae of the respiratory system and gastrointestinal system the bird may show ophthalmic signs and refuse to drink.

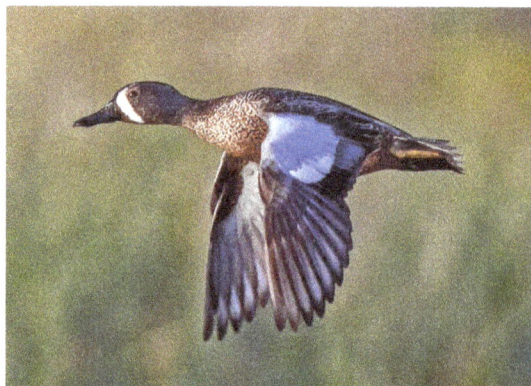

Blue winged teal can be infected by DEV, but are one of the least susceptible species

Anatid alphaherpesvirus 1 can only infect birds of the *Anseriformes* order and *Anatidae* family, with the possible exception of coots. A study of lesions found in "coots (order *Gruiformes*)" found similarities to DEV lesions. This could be evidence that DEV is able to "cross to different orders and families" or "adapted to new hosts." Waterfowl species have differing susceptibility to DEV, with wild fowl tending to be more resistant. Nonwaterfowl have not been shown to be infected by duck plague. Blue-winged teal have been found to be one the most susceptible species and mallards one of the least. In another it took 300,000 more virus material to infect northern pintail than to infect blue-winged teal.

Diagnosis can usually be made based on the clinical signs and postmortem findings:

> On post-mortem, petechial haemorrhage in the conjunctivae, mucous membranes, trachea, syrinx and intestine are pathognomonic for DEV. Diagnosis can also be confirmed with presence of virus inclusion bodies in tissues or a positive immunohistochemical staining for viral antigen.

Epidemiology

DEV is found during the spring seasons across the globe. The United States, Netherlands, and UK have the most occurrences from March to June. Whereas, Southern Hemisphere populations, such as in Brazil, are more likely to have outbreaks November through February during their spring season.

If host organisms survive primary infection, they enter a latent stage lasting up to 4 years. Latent stage leads to vertical and horizontal transmission of DEV. Virus particles can be shed by the latent host in shared water or through direct contact (horizontal transmission), contributing to on-going epizootics. There is also evidence of vertical transmission from latent host carriers to their eggs and offspring, which will also be asymptomatic. However, during times of stress AHV-1 may move to nerve roots from nerve ganglia and "induce herpetic lesions", a visible symptom of latency carrying. Environmental and physiological cues cause latent carriers to shed viral particles. Examples of physiological cues include "stress of migration, breeding season, [and] social interaction." Primary latency sites in carries are the trigeminal ganglion, lymphoid tissue, and blood lymphocytes. The latency sites of APV-1 is similar to other herpesviruses.

Treatment and Control

Vaccination for duck viral enteritis is now routine in the United States. Only attenuated vaccines are efficacious. Once DEV is present, depopulation, relocation and intensive disinfection are required to overcome an outbreak. Solid natural immunity develops in recovered birds. There is no treatment for DEV, but resveratrol has shown to have some antiviral activity against the virus.

Management practices such as preventing exposure to wild waterfowl and contaminated water and screening of new stock should be performed to prevent disease.

Pathogenesis

DEV is considered pantropic because it is able to replicate and spread to multiple organs within the host. Viral replication causes an increase in vascular permeability, which leads to the lesions and hemorrhaging of organs, namely the liver, spleen, thymus, and bursa of Fabricius. DVH-1 replicates in the mucus membranes of bird's esophagus and cloaca, the two primary entrances of the virus. The means of infection influences which tissues will be affected first and the incubation time before symptoms show. Typically viral replication begins in the digestive track and moves to bursa of Fabricuis, thymus, spleen, and liver.

Virology

Classification

Anatid alphaherpesvirus 1 is under the *Herpesvirales* order, the *Herpesviridae* family, the *Alphaherpesvirinae* subfamily. The genus was identified as *Mardivirus*. Genomic evidence shows that APV-1 is genetically similar to *Human alphaherpesvirus 1* and *2* (HSV-1 and HSV-1), *Suid alphaherpesvirus 1*, *Equid alphaherpesvirus 1* and *4* (EHV-1 and EHV-4), and *Bovine alphaherpesvirus 1* (BHV-1).

Genome

Anatid alphaherpesvirus 1, similar to other herpesviruses, has a linear double stranded DNA genome. The dsDNA weight is 119×10^6 Daltons and approximately 158,091 base pairs long. AHV-1 has 67 genes in its genome, 65 of which are likely coding genes. Three of the genes have no homologs to other herpesviruses, and are unique to AHV-1. Unique long (UL), unique (US), unique short internal repeat (IRS), and unique short terminal repeat (TRS) regions make up the genome. The genomic arrangement is ordered as UL-IRS-US-TRS. There are 78 predicted proteins encoded by the genome.

Structure

DEV has similar morphology to other *Herpesvirales* viruses. Common elements of herpviruses include a "DNA core, icosahedral capsid, tegument, and envelope." The nucleocapsid of HPV-1 is 75 micrometers wide and the envelope diameter is 181 micrometers.

Replication and Transcription Cycle

Three phases (immediate early (IE), early (E), and late (L)) of infection dictate the transcription of certain DEV genes. Immediate early begins after infection and before viral DNA replication. During this phase IE genes are transcribed without other proteins. The E genes are also transcribed before viral DNA replication, but are dependent on the IE gene products. After entering the host organism a virion begins the process of replication by first attaching to cells using glycoprotein spikes. gB, gC, gD, gH, and gL are known to be involved. Similar Alphaviruses use gC protein to aid in binding the virion to the cell and gD to stabilize it, if required. gB, gD, gH, and gL proteins allow for fusion of the cell and envelope, and are necessary for survival.

Entrance to host cells begins infection, and is largely controlled by the US 2 viral protein. Envelope fusion with the plasma membrane of the host cell causes separation of the nucleocapsid from viral DNA and proteins. Multiple necessary viral proteins are located within the envelope. DNA and proteins enter the host cell nucleus and turn-off host cell synthesis of nucleic acids, proteins, and other macro molecules. There are two hypothesized origins of replication in the IRS and TRS regions of the genome. Immature capsids are formed from coiled DNA. L genes are transcribed "after the synthesis of DNA and viral protein onset." Virion DNA maturation occurs as the nucleocapids "bud through nuclear membrane." Completed viral replication occurs within 12 hours of infection. Vacuoles of mature virions are formed and released via exocytosis to other cells. Epithelial, lymphocytes, and macrophages are the favored sites of replication in the host organism.

Bovine Viral Diarrhea

Bovine viral diarrhea (BVD) or bovine viral diarrhoea (UK English), and previously referred to as bovine virus diarrhoea (BVD), is a significant economic disease of cattle that is endemic in the majority of countries throughout the world. Worldwide reviews of the economically assessed production losses and intervention programs (e.g. eradication programs, vaccination strategies and biosecurity measures) incurred by BVD infection have been published. The causative agent, bovine viral diarrhea virus (BVDV), is a member of the genus *Pestivirus* of the family Flaviviridae.

BVD infection results in a wide variety of clinical signs, due to its immunosuppressive effects, as well as having a direct effect on respiratory disease and fertility. In addition, BVD infection of a susceptible dam during a certain period of gestation can result in the production of a persistently infected (PI) fetus.

PI animals recognise intra-cellular BVD viral particles as 'self' and shed virus in large quantities throughout life; they represent the cornerstone of the success of BVD as a disease.

Currently, it was shown in a worldwide review study that the PI prevalence at animal level ranged from low ($\leq$0.8% Europe, North America, Australia), medium (>0.8% to 1.6% East Asia) to high (>1.6% West Asia). Countries that had failed to implement any BVDV control and/or eradication programmes (including vaccination) had the highest PI prevalence.

Virus Classification and Structure

BVDV is a member of the genus *Pestivirus*, belonging to the family *Flaviviridae*. Border disease virus (sheep) and classical swine fever virus (pigs) are other members of this genus that also cause significant financial loss to the livestock industry. Pestiviruses are small, spherical, single-stranded, enveloped RNA viruses of 40 to 60 nm in diameter. The genome consists of a single, linear, positive-sense, single-stranded RNA molecule of approximately 12.3 kb.

Two BVDV genotypes are recognised, based on the nucleotide sequence of the 5'untranslated (UTR) region; BVDV-1 and BVDV-2. BVDV-1 isolates have been grouped into 16 subtypes (a –p) and BVDV-2 has currently been grouped into 3 subtypes (a – c).

BVDV strains can be further divided into distinct biotypes (cytopathic or non-cytopathic) according to their effects on tissue cell culture; cytopathic (cp) biotypes, formed via mutation of non-cytopathic (ncp) biotypes, induce apoptosis in cultured cells. Ncp viruses can induce persistent infection in cells and have an intact NS2/3 protein. In cp viruses the NS2/3 protein is either cleaved to NS2 and NS3 or there is a duplication of viral RNA containing an additional NS3 region. The majority of BVDV infections in the field are caused by the ncp biotype.

Epidemiology

BVD is considered one of the most significant infectious diseases in the livestock industry world-wide due to its high prevalence, persistence and clinical consequences.

In Europe the prevalence of antibody positive animals in countries without systematic BVD control is between 60 and 80%. Prevalence has been determined in individual countries and tends to be positively associated with stocking density of cattle.

BVDV-1 strains are predominant in most parts of the world, whereas BVDV-2 represents 50% of cases in North America. In Europe, BVDV-2 was first isolated in the UK in 2000 and currently represents up to 11% of BVD cases in Europe.

Transmission of BVDV occurs both horizontally and vertically with both persistently and transiently infected animals excreting infectious virus. Virus is transmitted via direct contact, bodily secretions and contaminated fomites, with the virus being able to persist in the environment for more than two weeks. Persistently infected animals are the most important source of the virus, continuously excreting a viral load one thousand times that shed by acutely infected animals.

Pathogenesis

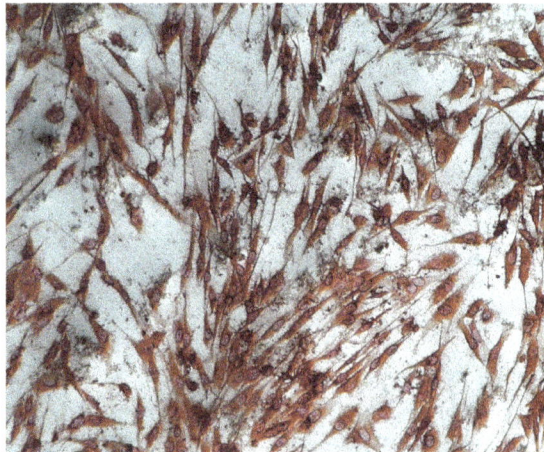

Turbinate cells infected with BVDV

Acute Transient Infection

Following viral entry and contact with the mucosal lining of the mouth or nose, replication occurs in epithelial cells. BVDV replication has a predilection for the palatine tonsils, lymphoid tissues and epithelium of the oropharynx.

Phagocytes take up BVDV or virus-infected cells and transport them to peripheral lymphoid tissues; the virus can also spread systemically through the bloodstream. Viraemia occurs 2–4 days after exposure and virus isolation from serum or leukocytes is generally possible between 3–10 days post infection.

During systemic spread the virus is able to gain entry into most tissues with a preference for lymphoid tissues. Neutralising antibodies can be detected from 10–14 days post infection with titres continuing to increase slowly for 8–10 weeks. After 2–3 weeks, antibodies effectively neutralise viral particles, promote clearance of virus and prevent seeding of target organs.

Intrauterine Infections

Fetal infection is of most consequence as this can result in the birth of a persistently infected neonate. The effects of fetal infection with BVDV are dependent upon the stage of gestation at which the dam suffers acute infection.

BVDV infection of the dam prior to conception, and during the first 18 days of gestation, results in delayed conception and an increased calving to conception interval. Once the embryo is attached, infection from days 29–41 can result in embryonic infection and resultant embryonic death.

Infection of the dam from approximately day 30 of gestation until day 120 can result in immunotolerance and the birth of calves persistently infected with the virus.

BVDV infection between 80 and 150 days of gestation may be teratogenic, with the type of birth defect dependent upon the stage of fetal development at infection. Abortion may occur at any time during gestation. Infection after approximately day 120 can result in the birth of a normal fetus which is BVD antigen-negative and BVD antibody-positive. This occurs because the fetal immune system has developed, by this stage of gestation, and has the ability to recognise and fight off the invading virus, producing anti-BVD antibodies.

Chronic Infections

BVD virus can be maintained as a chronic infection within some immunoprivileged sites following transient infection. These sites include ovarian follicles, testicular tissues, central nervous system and white blood cells. Cattle with chronic infections elicit a significant immune response, exhibited by extremely high antibody titres.

Clinical Signs

BVDV infection has a wide manifestation of clinical signs including fertility issues, milk drop, pyrexia, diarrhoea and fetal infection. Occasionally, a severe acute form of BVD may occur. These outbreaks are characterized by thrombocytopenia with high morbidity and mortality. However, clinical signs are frequently mild and infection insidious, recognised only by BVDV's immunosuppressive effects perpetuating other circulating infectious diseases (particularly scours and pneumonias).

PI Animals

Persistently infected animals did not have a competent immune system at the time of BVDV transplacental infection. The virus therefore entered the fetal cells and, during immune system development, was accepted as self. In PIs the virus remains present in a large number of the animal's body cells throughout its life and is continuously shed. PIs are often ill-thrifty and smaller than their peers, however they can appear normal. PIs are more susceptible to disease, with only 20% of PIs surviving to two years of age. If a PI dam is able to reproduce they always give birth to PI calves.

Mucosal Disease

The PI cattle that do survive ill-thrift are susceptible to mucosal disease. Mucosal disease only develops in PI animals and is invariably fatal. Disease results when a PI animal is superinfected with a cytopathic biotype arising from mutation of the non-cytopathic strain of BVDV already circulating in that animal. The cp BVDV spreads to the gastro-intestinal epithelium, and necrosis of keratinocytes results in erosion and ulceration. Fluid leaks from the epithelial surface of the gastro-intestinal tract causing diarrhoea and dehydration. In addition, bacterial infection of the damaged epithelium results in secondary septicaemia. Death occurs in the ensuing days or weeks.

Diagnosis

Various diagnostic tests are available for the detection of either active infection or evidence of historical infection. The method of diagnosis used also depends upon whether the vet is investigating at an individual or a herd level.

Virus or Antigen Detection

Antigen ELISA and rtPCR are currently the most frequently performed tests to detect virus or viral antigen. Individual testing of ear tissue tag samples or serum samples is performed. It is vital that repeat testing is performed on positive samples to distinguish between acute, transiently infected cattle and PIs. A second positive result, acquired at least three weeks after the primary result, indicates a PI animal. rtPCR can also be used on bulk tank milk (BTM) samples to detect any PI cows contributing to the tank. It is reported that the maximum number of contributing cows from which a PI can be detected is 300.

BVD Antibody Detection

Antibody (Ig) ELISAs are used to detect historical BVDV infection; these tests have been validated in serum, milk and bulk milk samples. Ig ELISAs do not diagnose active infection but detect the presence of antibodies produced by the animal in response to viral infection. Vaccination also induces an antibody response, which can result in false positive results, therefore it is important to know the vaccination status of the herd or individual when interpreting results. A standard test to assess whether virus has been circulating recently is to perform an Ig ELISA on blood from 5–10 young stock that have not been vaccinated, aged between 9 and 18 months. A positive result indicates exposure to BVDV, but also that any positive animals are very unlikely to be PI animals themselves. A positive result in a pregnant female indicates that she has previously been either vaccinated or infected with BVDV and could possibly be carrying a PI fetus, so antigen testing of the newborn is vital to rule this out. A negative antibody result, at the discretion of the responsible veterinarian, may require further confirmation that the animal is not in fact a PI.

At a herd level, a positive Ig result suggests that BVD virus has been circulating or the herd is vaccinated. Negative results suggest that a PI is unlikely however this naïve herd is in danger of severe consequences should an infected animal be introduced. Antibodies from wild infection or vaccination persist for several years therefore Ig ELISA testing is more valuable when used as a surveillance tool in seronegative herds.

Eradication and Control

The mainstay of eradication is the identification and removal of persistently infected animals. Re-infection is then prevented by vaccination and high levels of biosecurity, supported by continuing surveillance. PIs act as viral reservoirs and are the principal source of viral infection but transiently infected animals and contaminated fomites also play a significant role in transmission.

Leading the way in BVD eradication, almost 20 years ago, were the Scandinavian countries. Despite different conditions at the start of the projects in terms of legal support, and regardless of initial prevalence of herds with PI animals, it took all countries approximately 10 years to reach their final stages.

Once proven that BVD eradication could be achieved in a cost efficient way, a number of regional programmes followed in Europe, some of which have developed into national schemes.

Vaccination is an essential part of both control and eradication. While BVD virus is still circulating within the national herd, breeding cattle are at risk of producing PI neonates and the economic consequences of BVD are still relevant. Once eradication has been achieved, unvaccinated animals will represent a naïve and susceptible herd. Infection from imported animals or contaminated fomites brought into the farm, or via transiently infected in-contacts will have devastating consequences.

Vaccination

Modern vaccination programmes aim not only to provide a high level of protection from clinical disease for the dam, but, crucially, to protect against viraemia and prevent the production of PIs. While the immune mechanisms involved are the same, the level of immune protection required for foetal protection is much higher than for prevention of clinical disease.

While challenge studies indicate that killed, as well as live, vaccines prevent foetal infection under experimental conditions, the efficacy of vaccines under field conditions has been questioned. The birth of PI calves into vaccinated herds suggests that killed vaccines do not stand up to the challenge presented by the viral load excreted by a PI in the field.

Bird Flu

Bird flu, or avian influenza, is a viral infection spread from bird to bird. Currently, a particularly deadly strain of bird flu - H5N1 - continues to spread among poultry in Egypt and in certain parts of Asia.

Technically, H5N1 is a highly pathogenic avian influenza (HPAI) virus. It's deadly to most birds. And it's deadly to humans and to other mammals that catch the virus from birds. Since the first human case in 1997, H5N1 has killed nearly 60% of the people who have been infected.

But unlike human flu bugs, H5N1 bird flu does not spread easily from person to person. The very few cases of human-to-human transmission have been among people with exceptionally close contact, such as a mother who caught the virus while caring for her sick infant.

Migrating water fowl - most notably wild ducks - are the natural carriers of bird flu viruses. It's suspected that infection can spread from wild fowl to domestic poultry.

Because the disease has spread to wild birds, pigs, and even to donkeys, it will be difficult, if not impossible, to eradicate. As of 2011, the disease was well established in six nations: Bangladesh, China, Egypt, India, Indonesia, and Vietnam.

Infectious Bursal Disease

Infectious bursal disease, IBD (also known as Gumboro disease, infectious bursitis and infectious avian nephrosis) is a highly contagious disease of young chickens caused by infectious bursal disease virus (IBDV), characterized by immunosuppression and mortality generally at 3 to 6 weeks of age. The disease was first discovered in Gumboro, Delaware in 1962. It is economically important to the poultry industry worldwide due to increased susceptibility to other diseases and negative interference with effective vaccination. In recent years, very virulent strains of IBDV (vvIBDV), causing severe mortality in chicken, have emerged in Europe, Latin America, South-East Asia, Africa and the Middle East. Infection is via the oro-fecal route, with affected bird excreting high levels of the virus for approximately 2 weeks after infection.

Virology

IBDV is a double stranded RNA virus that has a bi-segmented genome and belongs to the genus *Avibirnavirus* of family *Birnaviridae*. There are two distinct serotypes of the virus, but only serotype 1 viruses cause disease in poultry. At least six antigenic subtypes of IBDV serotype 1 have been identified by *in vitro* cross-neutralization assay. Viruses belonging to one of these antigenic subtypes are commonly known as variants, which were reported to break through high levels of maternal antibodies in commercial flocks, causing up to 60 to 100 percent mortality rates in chickens. With the advent of highly sensitive molecular techniques, such as reverse transcription polymerase chain reaction (RT-PCR) and restriction fragment length polymorphism (RFLP), it became possible to detect the vvIBDV, to differentiate IBDV strains, and to use such information in studying the molecular epidemiology of the virus.

IBDV genome consists of two segments, A and B, which are enclosed within a nonenveloped icosahedral capsid. The genome segment B (2.9 kb) encodes VP1, the putative viral RNA polymerase. The larger segment A (3.2 kb) encodes viral proteins VP2, VP3, VP4, and VP5. Among them, VP2 protein contains important neutralizing antigenic sites and elicits protective immune response and most of the amino acid (AA) changes between antigenically different IBDVs are clustered in the hypervariable region of VP2. Thus, this hypervariable region of VP2 is the obvious target for the molecular techniques applied for IBDV detection and strain variation studies.

Viral Structure

The IBDV capsid protein exhibits structural domains that show homology to those of the capsid proteins of some positive-sense single-stranded RNA viruses, such as the nodaviruses and tetraviruses, as well as the T=13 capsid shell protein of the *Reoviridae*. The T=13 shell of the IBDV capsid is formed by trimers of VP2, a protein generated by removal of the C-terminal domain from its precursor, pVP2. The trimming of pVP2 is performed on immature particles as part of the maturation process. The other major structural protein, VP3, is a multifunctional component lying under the T=13 shell that influences the inherent structural polymorphism of pVP2. The virus-encoded RNA-dependent RNA polymerase, VP1, is incorporated into the capsid through its association with VP3. VP3 also interacts extensively with the viral dsRNA genome.

Pathogenesis

Clinical disease is associated to bird age with the greatest bursal mass, which occurs between 3 and 6 weeks of age. The greatest bursal mass is mostly a result of a large population of maturing IgM-bearing B-lymphocytes (lymphoblasts), the main target of infection. Young birds at around two to eight weeks of age that have highly active bursa of Fabricius are more susceptible to disease. Birds over eight weeks are resistant to challenge and will not show clinical signs unless infected by highly virulent strains.

Subclinical disease occurs in chickens infected before three weeks of age. At this age the B-lymphoblast population is smaller and the systemic effects are insufficient for generating clinical signs. However, the B-cell destruction is usually most severe in subclinically infected young, as virus will destroy a smaller population and most cells in one place (the bursa).

After ingestion, the virus destroys the lymphoid follicles in the bursa of Fabricius as well as the circulating B-cells in the secondary lymphoid tissues such as GALT (gut-associated lymphoid tissue), CALT (conjunctiva), BALT (Bronchial) caecal tonsils, Harderian gland, etc. Acute disease and death is due to the necrotizing effect of these viruses on the host tissues. Kidney failure is a common cause of mortality. If the bird survives and recovers from this phase of the disease, it remains immunocompromised which means it is more susceptible to other diseases.

Clinical Signs

Disease may appear suddenly and morbidity typically reaches 100%. In the acute form birds are prostrated, debilitated and dehydrated. They produce a watery diarrhea and may have swollen feces-stained vent. Most of the flock is recumbent and have ruffled feathers. Mortality rates vary with virulence of the strain involved, the challenge dose, previous immunity, presence of concurrent disease, as well as the flock's ability to mount an effective immune response. Immunosuppression of very young chickens, less than three weeks of age, is possibly the most important outcome and may not be clinically detectable (subclinical). In addition, infection with less virulent strains may not show overt clinical signs, but birds that have bursal atrophy with fibrotic or cystic follicles and lymphocytopenia before six weeks of age, may be susceptible to opportunistic infection and may die of infection by agents that would not usually cause disease in immunocompetent birds.

Diagnosis

A preliminary diagnosis can usually be made based on flock history, clinical signs and *post-mortem* (necropsy) examinations. However, definitive diagnosis can only be achieved by the specific detection and/or isolation and characterization of IBDV. Immunofluorescence or immunohistochemistry tests, based on anti-IBDV labelled antibodies, or in-situ hybridization, based on labelled complementary cDNA sequence probe, are useful for the specific detection of IBDV in infected tissues. RT-PCR was designed for the detection of IBDV genome, such as VP1 coding gene, with the possibility of PCR product sequences be determined for genetically comparing isolates and producing phylogenetic trees. Serological tests such as agar gel precipitation and ELISA, for detecting antibodies, are used for monitoring vaccine responses and might be additional information for diagnosis of infection of unvaccinated flocks.

Necropsy examination will usually show changes in the bursa of Fabricius such as swelling, oedema, haemorrhage, the presence of a jelly serosa transudate and eventually, bursal atrophy. Pathological changes, especially haemorrhages, may also be seen in the skeletal muscle, intestines, kidney and spleen.

Treatment and Control

Peri-focal vaccination may not be effective for the combat of an outbreak, due to the rapidity of wild-IBDV spreading.

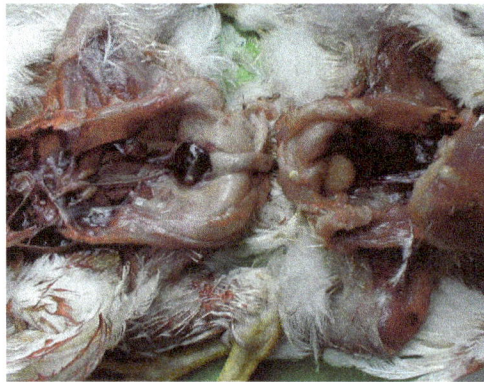

Two enlarged bursae: yellowish grey (right) and haemorrhagic (left)

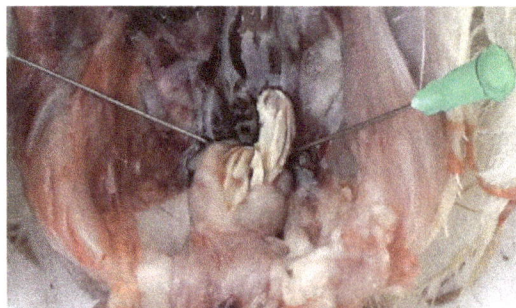

Caseous exudate in bursa of Fabricius

Passive immunity may protect against challenge with homologous IBDV, as does previous infection with homologous avirulent strains. Breeder flocks may be immunised against IBD so that they would transfer protective antibodies to their progenies, such as broiler and pullet chicks. Low-attenuated vaccine strains may cause damage to the bursa of Fabricius and immunosuppression in susceptible chicks. Biosecurity with adequate restriction to farm visitation and distancing from other flocks. Post outbreak hygiene measures may not be effective as the virus can survive for long periods in both housing and water.

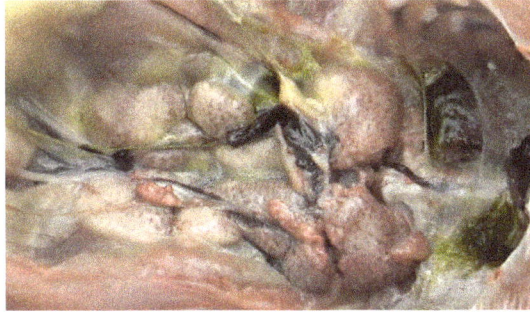

Lesions of kidneys

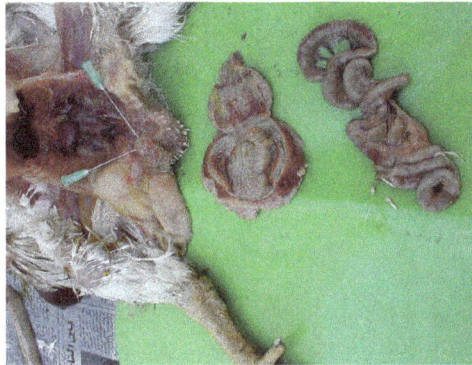

Haemorrhages in proventriculus and gizzard

Bovine Spongiform Encephalopathy

Bovine spongiform encephalopathy (BSE), commonly known as mad cow disease, is a neurode-generative disease of cattle. Symptoms include abnormal behavior, trouble walking, and weight loss. Later in the course the cow becomes unable to move. The time between infection and onset of symptoms is generally four to five years. Time from onset of symptoms to death is generally weeks to months. Spread to humans is believed to result in variant Creutzfeldt–Jakob disease (vCJD). As of 2018, a total of 231 cases of vCJD have been reported globally.

BSE is thought to be due to an infection by a misfolded protein, known as a prion. Cattle are believed to have been infected by being fed meat-and-bone meal (MBM) that contained the remains of cattle who spontaneously developed the disease or scrapie-infected sheep products. The outbreak increased throughout the United Kingdom due to the practice of feeding meat-and-bone meal to young calves of dairy cows. Cases are suspected based on symptoms and confirmed by examination of the brain. Cases are classified as classic or atypical, with the latter divided into H- and L types. It is a type of transmissible spongiform encephalopathy (TSE).

Efforts to prevent the disease in the UK include not allowing any animal older than 30 months to enter either the human food or animal feed supply. In Europe all cattle over 30 months must be tested if they will become human food. In North America tissue of concern, known as specified risk material, may not be added to animal feed or pet food. About 4.4 million cows were killed during the eradication program in the UK.

Four cases were reported globally in 2017, and the condition has been deemed to be nearly eradicated. In the United Kingdom, from 1986 to 2015, more than 184,000 cattle were diagnosed with the peak of new cases occurring in 1993. A few thousand additional cases have been reported in other regions of the world. It is believed that a few million cattle with the condition likely entered the food supply during the outbreak.

Signs

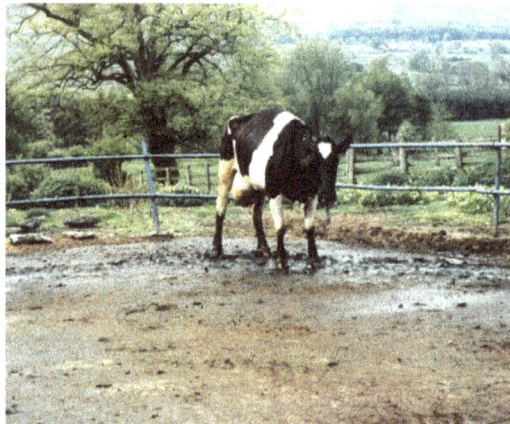

This cow with BSE displays abnormal posturing and weight loss

Signs are not seen immediately in cattle, due to the disease's extremely long incubation period. Some cattle have been observed to have an abnormal gait, changes in behavior, tremors and hyper-responsiveness to certain stimuli. Hindlimb ataxia affects the animal's gait and occurs when muscle control is lost. This results in poor balance and coordination. Behavioural changes may include aggression, anxiety relating to certain situations, nervousness, frenzy or an overall change in temperament. Some rare but previously observed signs also include persistent pacing, rubbing or licking. Additionally, nonspecific signs have also been observed which include weight loss, decreased milk production, lameness, ear infections and teeth grinding due to pain. Some animals may show a combination of these signs, while others may only be observed demonstrating one of the many reported. Once clinical signs arise, they typically get worse over the subsequent weeks and months, eventually leading to recumbency, coma and death.

Cause

BSE is an infectious disease believed to be due to a misfolded protein, known as a prion. Cattle are believed to have been infected from being fed meat and bone meal (MBM) that contained the remains of other cattle who spontaneously developed the disease or scrapie-infected sheep products. The outbreak increased throughout the United Kingdom due to the practice of feeding meat-and-bone meal to young calves of dairy cows.

Prions replicate by causing other normally folded proteins of the same type to take on their misfolded shape, which then go on to do the same, leading to an exponential chain reaction. Eventually, the prions aggregate into an alpha helical, beta pleated sheet, which is thought to be toxic to brain cells.

The agent is not destroyed even if the beef or material containing it is cooked or heat-treated.

Transmission can occur when healthy animals come in contact with tainted tissues from others with the disease. In the brain, the agent causes native cellular prion protein to deform into the misfolded state, which then goes on to deform further prion protein in an exponential cascade. This results in protein aggregates, which then form dense plaque fibers. Brain cells begin to die off in massive numbers, eventually leading to the microscopic appearance of "holes" in the brain, degeneration of physical and mental abilities, and ultimately death.

The British Government enquiry took the view that the cause was not scrapie, as had originally been postulated, but was some event in the 1970s that was not possible to identify.

Spread to Humans

Spread to humans is believed to result in variant Creutzfeldt–Jakob disease (vCJD). The agent can be transmitted to humans by eating food contaminated with it. The highest risk to humans is believed to be from eating food contaminated with the brain, spinal cord, or digestive tract though any tissue may be involved.

Pathogenesis

The pathogenesis of BSE is not well understood or documented like other diseases of this nature. Even though BSE is a disease that results in neurological defects, its pathogenesis occurs in areas that reside outside of the nervous system. There was a strong deposition of PrP^{Sc} initially located in the Ileal Peyer's patches of the small intestine. The lymphatic system has been identified in the pathogenesis of scrapie. It has not, however, been determined to be an essential part of the pathogenesis of BSE. The Ileal Peyer's patches have been the only organ from this system that has been found to play a major role in the pathogenesis. Infectivity of the Ileal Peyer's patches has been observed as early as 4 months after inoculation. PrP^{Sc} accumulation was found to occur mostly in tangible body macrophages of the Ileal Peyer's patches. Tangible body macrophages involved in PrP^{Sc} clearance are thought to play a role in PrP^{Sc} accumulation in the Peyer's patches. Accumulation of PrP^{Sc} was also found in follicular dendritic cells; however, it was of a lesser degree. Six months after inoculation, there was no infectivity in any tissues, only that of the ileum. This led researchers to believe that the disease agent replicates here. In naturally confirmed cases, there have been no reports of infectivity in the Ileal Peyer's patches. Generally, in clinical experiments, high doses of the disease are administered. In natural cases, it was hypothesized that low doses of the agent were present, and therefore, infectivity could not be observed.

Diagnosis

Diagnosis of BSE continues to be a practical problem. It has an incubation period of months to years, during which no signs are noticed, though the pathway of converting the normal brain prion protein (PrP) into the toxic, disease-related PrP^{Sc} form has started. At present, virtually no way is known to detect PrP^{Sc} reliably except by examining *post mortem* brain tissue using neuropathological and immunohistochemical methods. Accumulation of the abnormally folded PrP^{Sc} form of PrP is a characteristic of the disease, but it is present at very low levels in easily accessible body fluids such as blood or urine. Researchers have tried to develop methods to measure PrP^{Sc}, but no methods for use in materials such as blood have been accepted fully.

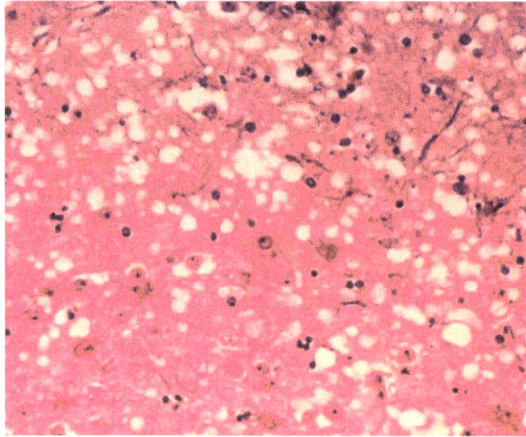

Brain tissue of a cow with BSE showing the typical microscopic "holes" in the grey matter

The traditional method of diagnosis relies on histopathological examination of the medulla oblongata of the brain, and other tissues, *post mortem*. Immunohistochemistry can be used to demonstrate prion protein accumulation.

In 2010, a team from New York described detection of PrP^{Sc} even when initially present at only one part in a hundred billion (10^{-11}) in brain tissue. The method combines amplification with a novel technology called surround optical fiber immunoassay and some specific antibodies against PrP^{Sc}. After amplifying and then concentrating any PrP^{Sc}, the samples are labelled with a fluorescent dye using an antibody for specificity and then finally loaded into a microcapillary tube. This tube is placed in a specially constructed apparatus so it is totally surrounded by optical fibres to capture all light emitted once the dye is excited using a laser. The technique allowed detection of PrP^{Sc} after many fewer cycles of conversion than others have achieved, substantially reducing the possibility of artifacts, as well as speeding up the assay. The researchers also tested their method on blood samples from apparently healthy sheep that went on to develop scrapie. The animals' brains were analysed once any signs became apparent. The researchers could, therefore, compare results from brain tissue and blood taken once the animals exhibited signs of the diseases, with blood obtained earlier in the animals' lives, and from uninfected animals. The results showed very clearly that PrP^{Sc} could be detected in the blood of animals long before the signs appeared. After further development and testing, this method could be of great value in surveillance as a blood- or urine-based screening test for BSE.

Classification

BSE is a transmissible disease that primarily affects the central nervous system; it is a form of transmissible spongiform encephalopathy, like Creutzfeldt–Jakob disease and kuru in humans and scrapie in sheep, and chronic wasting disease in deer.

Prevention

A ban on feeding meat and bone meal to cattle has resulted in a strong reduction in cases in countries where the disease has been present. In disease-free countries, control relies on import control, feeding regulations, and surveillance measures.

In UK and US slaughterhouses, the brain, spinal cord, trigeminal ganglia, intestines, eyes, and tonsils from cattle are classified as specified risk materials, and must be disposed of appropriately.

An enhanced BSE-related feed ban is in effect in both the United States and Canada to help improve prevention and elimination of BSE.

Epidemiology

The tests used for detecting BSE vary considerably, as do the regulations in various jurisdictions for when, and which cattle, must be tested. For instance in the EU, the cattle tested are older (30 months or older), while many cattle are slaughtered younger than that. At the opposite end of the scale, Japan tests all cattle at the time of slaughter. Tests are also difficult, as the altered prion protein has very low levels in blood or urine, and no other signal has been found. Newer tests are faster, more sensitive, and cheaper, so future figures possibly may be more comprehensive. Even so, currently the only reliable test is examination of tissues during a necropsy.

As for vCJD in humans, autopsy tests are not always done, so those figures, too, are likely to be too low, but probably by a lesser fraction. In the United Kingdom, anyone with possible vCJD symptoms must be reported to the Creutzfeldt–Jakob Disease Surveillance Unit. In the United States, the CDC has refused to impose a national requirement that physicians and hospitals report cases of the disease. Instead, the agency relies on other methods, including death certificates and urging physicians to send suspicious cases to the National Prion Disease Pathology Surveillance Center (NPDPSC) at Case Western Reserve University in Cleveland, which is funded by the CDC.

To control potential transmission of vCJD within the United States, the American Red Cross has established strict restrictions on individuals' eligibility to donate blood. Individuals who have spent a cumulative time of 3 months or more in the United Kingdom between 1980 and 1996, or a cumulative time of 5 years or more from 1980 to present in any combination of countries in Europe, are prohibited from donating blood.

Rift Valley Fever

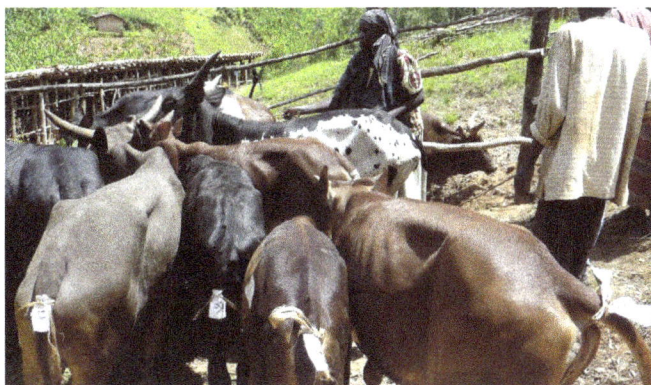

Rift Valley fever (RVF) is an acute, fever-causing viral disease most commonly observed in domesticated animals (such as cattle, buffalo, sheep, goats, and camels), with the ability to infect and cause illness in humans. The disease is caused by RVF virus (RVFV), a member of the genus Phlebovirus in the family Bunyaviridae. It was first reported in livestock by veterinary officers in Kenya's Rift Valley in the early 1910s.

RVF is generally found in regions of eastern and southern Africa where sheep and cattle are raised, but the virus exists in most of sub-Saharan Africa, including west Africa and Madagascar. In September 2000, a RVF outbreak was reported in Saudi Arabia and subsequently, Yemen. This outbreak represents the first cases of Rift Valley fever identified outside Africa.

Outbreaks of RVF can have major societal impacts, including significant economic losses and trade reductions. The virus most commonly affects livestock, causing disease and abortion in domesticated animals, an important income source for many. Outbreaks of disease in animal populations are called "epizootics." The most notable RVF epizootic occurred in Kenya in 1950-1951, resulting in the death of an estimated 100,000 sheep.

Additionally, epizootic outbreaks of RVF increase the likelihood of contact between diseased animals and humans, which can lead to epidemics of RVF in humans. One example occurred in 1977 when the virus was detected in Egypt (possibly imported from infected domestic animals from Sudan) and caused a large outbreak of RVF among both animals and humans resulting in over 600 human deaths. Another example of RVF spillover into human populations occurred in west Africa in 1987, and was linked to construction of the Senegal River Project. The project caused flooding in the lower Senegal River area, altering ecological conditions and interactions between animals and humans. As a result, a large RVF outbreak occurred in animals and humans.

Equine Influenza

Equine Infl uenza (EI) is a highly contagious though rarely fatal respiratory disease of horses, donkeys and mules and other equidae. The disease has been recorded throughout history, and when horses were the main draft animals, outbreaks of EI crippled the economy. Nowadays outbreaks still have a severe impact on the horse industry.

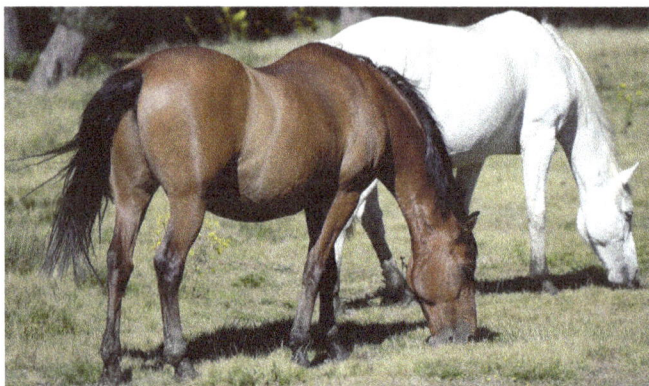

EI is caused by two subtypes of infl uenza A viruses: H7N7 and H3N8, of the family Orthomyxoviridae. They are related to but distinct from the viruses that cause human and avian infl uenza.

Equine Infl uenza is a disease listed in the OIE Terrestrial Animal Health Code and countries are obligated to report the occurrence of the disease according to the OIE Code.

The disease is entrenched in most of the world, with the exceptions of Australia (where an import-ant outbreak occurred in 2007), New Zealand, and Iceland.

Disease Transmitted and Spread

Highly contagious, EI is spread by contact with infected animals, which in coughing excrete the virus. In fact animals can begin to excrete the virus as they develop a fever before showing clinical signs. It can also be spread by mechanical transmission of the virus on clothing, equipment, brush-es etc carried by people working with horses.

Once introduced into an area with a susceptible population, the disease, with an incubation period of only one to three days, spreads quickly and is capable of causing explosive outbreaks. Crowding and transportation are factors that favour the spread of EI.

Clinical Signs of the Disease

In fully susceptible animals, clinical signs include fever and a harsh dry cough followed by a nasal discharge. Depression, loss of appetite, muscle pain and weakness are frequently observed. The clinical signs generally abate within a few days, but complications due to secondary infections are common. While most animals recover in two weeks, the cough may continue longer and it may take as much as six months for some horses to regain their full ability. If animals are not rested adequately, the clinical course is prolonged.

While the disease is rarely fatal, complications such as pneumonia are common, causing long term debility of horses, and death can occur due to pneumonia, especially in foals.

Disease Diagnosed

Clinical signs are suggestive of EI, but defi nitive diagnosis is by serology or isolation of the vi-rus according to procedures in the OIE Manual of Diagnostic Tests and Vaccines for Terrestrial Animals.

Prevent or Control the Disease

Vaccination is practiced in most countries. However, due to the variability of the strains of virus in circulation, and the diffi culty in matching the vaccine strain to the strains of virus in circulation, vaccination does not always prevent infection although it can reduce the severity of the disease and speed recovery times. The OIE also convenes an Expert Surveillance Panel on Equine Infl uenza Vaccine that examines the strains of virus in circulation making recommendations on which strains should be included in the vaccines.

When the disease appears, efforts are placed on movement control and isolation of infected horses. The virus is easily killed by common disinfectants, so thorough cleaning and disinfection is part of biosecurity measures in responding to the disease.

Since the disease is most often introduced by an infected animal, isolation of new entries to a farm or stable is paramount to preventing the introduction of disease to a premise.

For movement of horses across international boundaries the OIE Terrestrial Animal Health Code sets the standards by which countries should control the import of horses.

Public Health Risk Associated with this Disease

There is little risk to public health. In experimental settings the virus has shown the ability to infect humans, and a few people in contact with infected horses developed antibodies to equine influenza viruses, but no humans exposed to the virus have become ill.

Disease Prevention and Control Measures

Prevention of Environmental Contamination

- The premises (sheds, stables, and kennels) and pastures should be prevented from contamination.

- Elimination of parasites from the host at the most appropriate time by use of antiparasiticides thereby preventing pasture contamination.

- Destruction of adult parasites in hosts prevents expulsion of eggs or the larvae and the associated contamination of the environment.

- Ovicidal drugs should preferably be used to destroy the eggs, thereby preventing environmental contamination.

- Anthelmentic treatments prior to rainy seasons using larvicidal drugs will prevent contamination of pastures at a time when conditions are becoming favourable for egg and larval development.

- Proper faeces disposal will give satisfactory control of faecally transmitted monoxenous parasites of animals.

- Faeces or litter may be heaped to destroy the eggs/oocysts of parasites.

- Pens and pastures should not be overstocked.

- Reducing the stocking rate can significantly reduce the parasite burden in animals and the associated problem of contamination in sheds and pastures.

Control of Intermediate Host, Vectors and Reservoirs

- Limiting the contact between intermediate and final hosts by improvements in management.

- Direct action may be taken to reduce or eliminate intermediate host populations.

- Reduction in the number of snail intermediate host by chemical (molluscides) or biological control (ducks, Maris species of snails).

- Reduction in the number of snail intermediate hosts by drainage, fencing and other management practices.

- Reduction in the number of insect and tick vectors by chemical (insecticides/acaricides), biological control (hymenopterous insects, entomopathogenic fungi and Bacillus thuringiensis) and genetic control (sterile male technique, chromosomal translocation).

- Use of vaccines (Tickgard) at appropriate times may control the vector population.

- Destruction of reservoir hosts is important in controlling certain parasites, e.g., rodents for Leishmania and antelopes for African trypanosomes.

Control of Internal Parasites

- Ridding the animal of internal parasites by periodical deworming.

- Preventing infestation of animals by keeping premises free from infective forms of parasite disinfestations.

- Elimination of intermediate hosts.

Control of Arthropod Pests

- Manure, filth, damp and dark corners, stagnant water etc. are all favorite breeding places of insects and these places should be concentrated for removal and cleaning periodically.

- Eggs of ticks and mites deposited in cracks and crevices in the walls, floors and wood work of the animal houses should be removed periodically.

- Periodical (once in April-June and once in July-September) dipping or spraying of animals with suitable insecticides to prevent lice, flies, fleas, mites and ticks on skin of animals.

- Inside of animal sheds should be scrubbed and cleaned daily to remove all filth.

- Areas around animal sheds should also be kept dry and clean.

- Interior of animal sheds (roofs, walls and corners) should be cleared regularly of cobwebs and spider webs and sprayed with insecticides at least once in a month.

- Dusting of animals with DDT, lorexane, gammexane or with some patent preparations available in the market can be tried to control cattle warble flies, etc.

- If the herd is small, individual animals can be dusted by hand.

- For larger herds a gunny bag (or any other bag having sufficiently large pores through which dusting powder can escape out) filled with dusting powder can be hung at a convenient place and at a convenient place and at a convenient height. As the animals pass under the bag they rub their backs against the bag, getting a dusting in the process. Such convenient places for hanging the bags are the entrances to stanchion barn, hay or straw feeding bunk, gates leading out on to the pasture etc.

- Organophosphate insecticides like Malathion, Parathion, and Neguvon etc. are available which are very destructive to insects but are quite toxic to animals as well.

- Newer generation synthetic pyrethroids like Deltamethrin (ButoxTM), Cypermethrin (Cyprol, Tikkil) etc. are available in the market.

- Great care should be taken while using these chemicals and manufacturer's instructions regarding their usage should be scrupulously followed.

Control and Reducing the Infection as soon as an Outbreak Occurs

- Segregate sick animals.

- Stop all animals, animal products, vehicles and persons coming into and out of the farm.

- Call a veterinarian for advice, adopt containment vaccination.

- Avoid grazing in a common place.

- Ban all visitors to the farm.

- Provide foot dips containing disinfectants at the entry of the farm and gear up sanitation and hygiene.

Isolation of Sick Animals

- Isolation means segregation of animals, which are known to be or suspected to be affected with a contagious disease from the apparently healthy ones.

- Segregated animals should be housed in a separate isolation ward situated far away from the normal animal houses.

- The isolation ward should never be at a higher level than that of the healthy shed.

- If a separate accommodation is not available the animals concerned should be placed at one end of normal animals' buildings, as far away from healthy stock as practicable.

- Attendants working on sick animals and equipment such as buckets, shovels etc. used for them should not be used for healthy stock. If this is not practicable, the sick animals should be attended to daily, after the healthy stock. After this, the equipment should be thoroughly disinfected before they are used on healthy stock next day; the attendant too should wash his hands and feet in antiseptic and discard the clothes in which he worked. v The isolated animals should be brought back into the herd only when the outbreak ends and they are fully recovered.

Quarantine for Newly Purchased Animals

- Quarantine is the segregation of apparently healthy animals (especially animals being brought into the herd for the first time), which have been exposed to the risk of infection from those animals, which are healthy and unexposed to the risk of infection.

- The idea is to give sufficient time for any contagious disease that the quarantine animals may be having, to become active and obvious. Hence, the quarantined period depends on the incubation period of a disease. But in practice a quarantine period of 30 days covers almost all diseases.

- For rabies, the quarantine period should be about six months.

- During the quarantine period, animals should be thoroughly screened for parasitic infestation by faecal examination and de-worming carried out on the 23rd/24th day, if need be.

- The animals should also be subjected to dipping or spraying on the 25th/26th day for removing ectoparasites if any.

Vaccination of Farm Animals

- Vaccination is a practice of artificially building up in the animal body immunity against specific infectious diseases by injecting biological agents called vaccines.

- The term vaccine is used to denote an antigen (substance form organisms) consisting of a live, attenuated or dead bacterium, virus or fungus and used for the production of active immunity in animals.

- The term also includes substances like toxins, toxoids or any other metabolites etc. produced by microbes and used for vaccination.

- The farm animals and young ones should be vaccinated at regular intervals at appropriate times.

- Vaccination should be done with consultation of veterinarians.

Deworming of Animals

- It is essential to deworm livestock regularly.

- The individual farmer should also try to keep his herd worm-free.

- The most suitable time of deworming is the early stages of infection when the worm load is less.

- The local veterinarian should be consulted for all suggestions regarding dewormers and deworming.

- In adult animals deworming is done on examination of dung.

- It is good to deworm adult females after parturition.

- All the animals should preferably be fasted for 24 hours before giving the anthelmentic.

- Young animals should preferably be dewormed every month using a suitable anthelmentic.

- Older stock can be dewormed at 4-6 months' intervals. The National Dairy Research Institute, Karnal recommended the following deworming schedule for calves. Such a deworming schedule is very crucial for buffalo calves, in which species mortality due to worms is very high.

- In places where heavy endo-parasite infestations are found (hot-humid regions) it is advisable to deworm heifers twice a year up to two years of age.

- Even adult stock can be drenched twice a year-once before monsoon season (May-June) and once during monsoon (August-September).

Elimination of Carriers

- An animal recovers from a disease, although apparently in good health the causative organism harbors in its tissues. Such germ carrying animals are known as 'carriers'.

- The carrier state may remain for years and the animal becomes a potential danger to susceptible animals.

- Common diseases for which carriers have been observed in farm animals are Tuberculosis, Leptospirosis and Brucellosis.

- Carriers of diseases in the herd should be diagnosed and eliminated so that the herd may be completely free from diseases.

- Certain diagnostic screening tests can be used for spotting out carriers animals in the herd. These tests should be periodically conducted on all animals in the herd so that carriers can be diagnosed and culled.

- Some of the commonly used screening tests are tuberculin test, Johnin test, agglutination test and test for detection of subclinical mastitis.

Tuberculin Test

- On injection of tuberculin (purified protein derivatives (PPD) of Mycobacterium tuberculosis (tubercle bacteria)) into an infected animal, allergic symptoms are set up, and these constitute a 'reaction'.

- In healthy animals, tuberculin, even in large doses, gives no reaction. This is quite a reliable test for diagnosing non-clinical cases of tuberculosis in all species of farm animals.

- Tuberculin test should be carried out in animal farms once every six months in the initial stages and later on, depending on the health status of the herd, the test can be conducted annually.

- January is the ideal month for conducting tuberculin test under Indian conditions.

- The important methods of test are intradermal, subcutaneous and ophthalmic, the former being most practicable, reliable and popular.

- Intradermal test can be used in all bovines.

- The best site is the side of neck.

- In bovines it can also be done in one of the folds of the skin by raising the tail, or on the vulva.

- In the neck, the sites for the middle third of the neck, as sites near the shoulder or mandible give less pronounced reactions.

- A small area of skin is clipped and cleansed with spirit.

- 0.1 ml of PPD is injected intradermally. If correctly done, the tuberculin creates a bead-like swelling detectable by the finger.

- The positive carrier animals should be culled and destroyed from the herd.

Johnin Test

- Johnin is (purified protein derivative of Mycobacterium paratuberculosis (Johne's bacterium)) used as a diagnostic test for Johne's disease in cattle and buffaloes.

- Johnin test is also done like single intradermal test done for tuberculosis.

- A painful indurated skin with an increase in skin thickness more than 4 mm is taken as positive.

- All positive animals are culled and destroyed.

Agglutination Test for Brucellosis

- This is a serological test based on the principle of antigen (dead bacteria) and antibody (agglutinins present in the body fluids, mainly serum of infected animals) reaction, resulting in agglutination of bacteria.

- When the agglutinins present in the serum and other body fluids of animals suffering with brucellosis or carriers is added to a suspension of killed culture of Brucella abortus organisms, the latter will cluster together; the reaction being known as agglutination.

- Healthy animal in which agglutinins are absent, do not show such agglutinations.

- Rapid plate agglutination test, which can be done at the site of the animal.

- Standard Tube Agglutination Test, which can be done in a laboratory.

- Agglutination can be conducted using whole blood, serum, milk, whey, semen, etc.

- Stockmen can only attempt to collect sterile samples of blood (from jugular vein) or milk of their animals periodically (say once in a year) and get them tested in the nearest laboratory.

- All positive reactors to the test should promptly be eliminated from the herd.

- Test for mastitis-Strip Cup Test.

- Strip Cup test comprises of letting the first few streams of milk from each quarter on to the black disc of strip cup. This will show up any clots, which only occur in the fore-milk in mild cases of mastitis, and will permit early treatment.

- Addition of an anionic detergent (such as alkyl sulphates or sulphonates, Teepol) to mastitis milk results in formation of typical gel streaks or clumps, according to the degree of abnormality of milk.

Test for Mastitis-California Mastitis Test (CMT)

- Milk from each of the four quarters is drawn into separate cups within a plastic paddle fitted with a handle, the cups being marked A, B, C and D to correspond with the quarters so designated.

- By tilting the paddle to an almost vertical position, surplus milk is allowed to run over, leaving only desired quantity of about 2ml.

- To this is added approximately the same quantity of CMT reagent (sodium lauryl sulphate – 4g, Teepol – 15 ml, Distilled water – 100 ml, Bromocresol purple – 100 mg) from a plastic container, care being taken to avoid production of foam or bubbles.

- The milk and fluid are immediately mixed by rapid rotation of the paddle in a horizontal plane while the reactions are noted.

- Formation of typical streaks and clumps indicate mastitis; the severity of reaction roughly indicating intensity of mastitis.

- After the cups have been emptied into a container and the paddle rinsed in clear water (the detergent quality of the test fluid ensures rapid and good cleaning) the apparatus may immediately be used for the next test without drying.

- All the milch animals should be screened for mastitis by strip cup test or CMT test at least once in a month, preferably more frequently.

- The sub clinically positive animals should be isolated from the herd and treated immediately.

Disposal of Carcass

- Proper disposal of carcasses of animals died of infectious disease is of utmost importance in preventing the spread of diseases to other animals and humans.

- Carcasses should never be disposed off by depositing them in or near a stream of flowing water, because this will carry infections to points downstream.

- An animal died of a infectious disease should not be allowed to remain longer in sheds as biting insects, rodents, etc. can reach it.

- Unless approved by a veterinarian (even then, only in a disinfected place) it is not safe to open carcasses of animals that have died of a disease.

- All carcasses should be disposed of properly either by burying or by burning.

Burial of Carcass

- The most common method of carcass disposal is burial.

- This is a reasonably safe method if done deeply enough and in soil from which there is no drainage to neighboring places.

- Deep burial is necessary to prevent worms carrying bacterial spores to the surface as well as to prevent carnivorous animals from digging up the carcass.

- The carcass should be carried to the burial place in a trolley and never by dragging it over the ground.

- The burial pit should be got ready before the carcass is taken there.

- The pit should be so dug that the highest part of the carcass must be at least 1.5 m below the level of the land surface.

- Bedding used for the dead animals, its excreta, feed left over by it and the top 5 cm soil form where the dead animals was lying (if the floor is not cemented) should also be buried along with the carcass.

- Drainage of water out of the burial place can be checked by seeing to it that the burial place is an area where the general water level is at least 2.5 m below the ground.

- The carcass is then covered with a thick layer of freshly burnt quicklime and then filled with dirt and topped with some rocks, to further circumvent marauders.

Burning of Carcass

- The most sanitary method of destroying carcasses is to burn them, preferably close to the site of their death, without dragging them any more than is absolutely necessary; even then only in trolley. Site for burning having been decided upon, the trench should be dug.

- The trench should be at least 0.5m deep, shallower towards the ends, and comparing in width and length to the carcass's size. General direction of the trench should be that of the prevailing wing direction.

- The trench is first filled with wood, some iron bars placed across it and the carcass placed thereon. By firing the wood, the carcass will be completely consumed and, with it, all infectious material.

- In towns and cities the so-called carcass utilization or carcass frying or rendering plants are usually available for industrial utilization of animal's carcasses. In these the skins are removed with due regard for the dangers of disease dissemination. After removal, the skins are usually disinfected by immersion in a disinfecting solution and the remainder of the carcass 'fried out' for its fat, the latter being used in manufacture of soap. Farmers can inform these plants whenever there is a carcass so that these utilization plants can collect the same.

Disinfection of Animal Houses

- Under ordinary conditions, daily scrubbing and washing of houses and the action of sunlight falling in the houses are sufficient enough to keep them moderately germ-free.

- But when a disease outbreak has occurred disinfection is a must and should be carried out scrupulously.

- All floors, walls up to height of 1.5 m, interiors of mangers, water troughs and other fittings and equipments coming in contact with animals are all to be disinfected.

- The first step in disinfection of animal houses is removal of all filth, as the power of disinfectants is greatly reduced in the presence of organic matter.

- Floors, walls up to height of 1.5 m interior of water troughs and mangers should be well scrubbed and all dung, litter etc. should be removed and stacked separately, where animals cannot reach.

- In case of an outbreak of anthrax, the dung, litter etc. should first be disinfected in situ thorough sprinkling of suitable disinfectant. If the floor is of earth, which is generally the case in Indian villages, the top 10cm earth should be removed and disposed off along with litter.

- After removal of filth, the place should be scrubbed and washed with 4 per cent hot washing soda solution (i.e., 4 kg washing soda in 100 litres of boiling water).

- The approved disinfectant solution should then be coated liberally over the place by sprinkling or preferably by spraying and left so to act for 24 hours.

- After this period, the animal house should again be washed with clean water and left to dry by wind and sunlight.

- The interior of water troughs and mangers should be whitewashed. (This can be done even routinely at fortnightly intervals.)

Disinfection of Pastures

- Removal of any obvious infective material, like carcass, aborted foetus, dung etc. from over the pasture and prevention of animals from grazing on the pasture under question for at least three to four months.

- The pasture can be ploughed up and left fallow for about six months during which period the pathogens would be destroyed by sun.

Common Disinfectants and their usage

- Bleaching powder (Chloride of lime)

  ○ It can be used for disinfection of animal houses when a contagious disease has occurred and for sterilization of water supplies.

- It should not be used in milking barns as its strong odour may taint milk.

- Concentration required is not less than 30 per cent available chlorine.

- Mode of application is dusting.

- Bleaching powder must be stored in airtight bins as damp surroundings, exposure light and air causes it decompose rapidly.

- Boric acid

  - It can be used as an udder wash.

  - It is a week antiseptic and is likely to harm nervous system if absorbed into body in large quantities.

  - It is used as wash for eyes and other sensitive parts of body.

  - Concentration required is 6 per cent solution.

  - Mode of application is splashing.

  - Nowadays antibiotic solutions are replacing boric acid as eyewash solution.

- Caustic soda (Sodium hydroxide)

  - For general use in farm buildings and animal houses, caustic soda is a very effective disinfectant as it is an excellent cleaning agent as well as a powerful germicide.

  - It is highly destructive to virus of foot and mouth disease, hog cholera etc.

  - It is not effective against tuberculosis and johne's disease organisms.

  - Concentration required is 2 per cent solution for general use and 5 percent solution against spores of anthrax and black quarter.

  - Mode of application is splashing.

  - Rubber gloves, goggles and protective clothing should always be worn when caustic soda solution is being used as it burns skin and damages fabrics.

- Cresols

  - The cresols are only slightly soluble in water and are therefore generally emulsified with soap.

  - Effective against a wide range of organisms including acid fast tuberculosis and Johne's disease bacteria but not effective against viruses and spores.

  - Good for disinfecting floors, walls, equipment etc. but not in milking barns because of its phenolic odour.

  - Concentration required is 2-3 per cent.

  - Mode of application is splashing.

- ○ Use only soft water for preparing solutions, hard water precipitates soap.

- ○ Lysol is a solution of cresol with soap.

- Lime (Calcium Oxide, quick lime)

  - ○ It is a deodorant as well as a disinfectant.

  - ○ It can be used for sprinkling on manure and animal discharges, on floors or as a white-wash or milk of lime (also known as slacked lime).

  - ○ Mode of application is sprinkling, scrubbing or sometimes dusting.

  - ○ Always use freshly prepared lime only.

- Phenol (Carbolic acid)

  - ○ Effective against several types of bacteria; not so effective on spores and viruses.

  - ○ Its disinfectant value is not reduced by the presence of organic matter but oil or alcohol does so.

  - ○ It is very toxic, corrosive and irritant.

  - ○ Concentration required is 1-2 per cent.

  - ○ Mode of application is splashing.

  - ○ Great care should be taken in using phenol to protect eyes, skin and clothing.

- Quaternary Ammonium Compounds (QAC)

  - ○ These are cationic detergents.

  - ○ They have no effect on spores and viruses.

  - ○ They can be used to disinfect dairy utensils, udders, milkers' hands and towels for wiping udders.

  - ○ Cetrimide, a white powder is an example for QAC.

  - ○ Concentration requires is 0.1 per cent solution (0.5 per cent cream for applying on teats and hands to prevent mastitis.

  - ○ Mode of application is wiping of udder with clothes wetted in 0.1 per cent solution; washing of milkers' hands.

  - ○ Utensils should be scrubbed with boiling water before rinsing with QAC.

- Soap

  - ○ Soap is an anionic detergent.

  - ○ It is a very week germicide.

- ° But its great usefulness in cleaning various surfaces including skin.

- ° It can be used preparatory to the application of a disinfectant.

- ° Mode of application is scrubbing.

- ° It should preferably be used only as surface-sanitizing agent.

- Sodium hypochlorite

  - ° It is a chlorine compound.

  - ° It is an excellent disinfectant but is not effective against T.B bacteria and its effectiveness is reduced by the presence of organic matter.

  - ° Concentration required is 200 parts per million of available chlorine about 300 ml sodium hypochlorite and about 200g of washing soda in 100 litres of hot water for washing utensils etc. For udder wash-about 60 ml in 10 litres of clean water.

  - ° Rinsing of utensils, wiping of udder.

  - ° Should be stored in air-tight containers as hypochlorites deteriorate rapidly when exposed to air.

- Washing Soda (Soda ash, Sodium carbonate)

  - ° It is good for disinfection of barn premises upon which an outbreak of virus disease like foot-and-mouth disease has occurred.

  - ° It is a good detergent.

  - ° Concentration required is 4 per cent solution.

  - ° Mode of application is scrubbing.

  - ° Lye is better against Foot-and-mouth disease virus than soda ash.

  - ° It should be used as a hot solution.

General Disease Prevention Measures

- Feed should be placed in troughs that cannot be contaminated by faeces and waterers should be kept clean and free of contaminants.

- Good grazing management will control pasture or grassland borne helminthic infections.

- Use of clean or safe pastures (not grazed for 6 to 12 months) will help to control helminths problems.

- Rotational grazing of livestock species should be followed to minimize or limit the infection from pasture.

- All new arrivals to the farm should be isolated for at least 30 days and dewormed.

- Young animals are generally more susceptible to parasites than adults. Therefore young animals should be housed separately from adult animals.

- Infected/Infested animals should be removed from the flock or herd and housed separately.

- Treatment should be followed by chemoprophylaxis to prevent reinfection.

- Vaccines may be used to prevent infection, if suitable vaccines are available.

- Prompt and proper disposal of manure and other filth from the farm premises.

- Regular scrubbing and cleaning of feed and water troughs as well as whitewashing their interior at least once in a week.

- Leveling up all ditches, low marshy areas, pits etc. in and around animal houses so that water may not stagnate in them.

- Filling up or fencing of all stagnant water pools, ponds etc. around the farm and on pastures so that animals may not get access to them. It is always better to have piped water supply to farm animals.

- Housing animals in clean houses with paved floors.

- Animals of different ages should be housed separately.

- Younger animals should never be mixed with older ones.

- Proper deworming of all such animals before putting them in a shed or bringing them into the farm.

- If grazing is practiced-division of pasture into several blocks and practicing rotational grazing in these blocks.

- Feeding of cultivated fodders is more helpful in checking pasture-borne infections.

- Preventing humans from defecating on pastures or around the farm, as this may cause contamination with tape worm eggs.

- Care should be taken to see that dogs (intermediate hosts), crows and other birds (mechanical carriers) do not gain access to the animal farm.

- Control of snail population may result in control of liver fluke infestation to some extent.

- It is worthwhile trying reduction of snail population by treating infected pastures, ponds, streams, etc. with copper sulphate.

- A concentration of one part of copper sulphate in one million parts of water is generally recommended but stronger solution may be necessary when large quantities of decaying organic matter are present.

References

- Mettenleiter (2008). "Molecular Biology of Animal Herpesviruses". Animal Viruses: Molecular Biology. Caister Academic Press. ISBN 978-1-904455-22-6

- Animal-disease, science: britannica.com, Retrieved 11 June, 2019

- Li, Yufeng; Huang, Bing; Ma, Xiuli; Wu, Jing; Li, Feng; Ai, Wu; Song, Minxun; Yang, Hanchun (2009). "Molecular characterization of the genome of duck enteritis virus". Virology. 391 (2): 151–161. doi:10.1016/j.virol.2009.06.018. PMID 19595405

- What-know-about-bird-flu, flu-guide, cold-and-flu: webmd.com, Retrieved 29 May, 2019

- Balasuriya, UB (December 2014). "Equine viral arteritis". The Veterinary Clinics of North America. Equine Practice. 30 (3): 543–60. doi:10.1016/j.cveq.2014.08.011. PMID 25441113

3
Zoonotic Diseases

The infectious diseases which spread from animals to humans are known as zoonotic diseases. They can be caused due to bacteria, viruses or parasites. Some of the common zoonotic diseases are anthrax, Ebola virus disease, rat-bite fever and rabies. This chapter closely examines these zoonotic diseases to provide an extensive understanding of the subject.

Zoonosis refers to diseases that can be passed from animals to humans. They are sometimes called zoonotic diseases.

Animals can carry harmful germs, such as bacteria, fungi, parasites, and viruses. These are then shared with humans and cause illness. Zoonotic diseases range from mild to severe, and some can even be fatal.

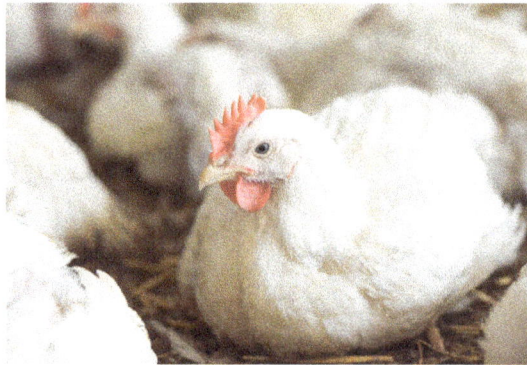

Many different types of animals may spread zoonotic diseases, including chickens

Zoonotic diseases are widespread both in the U.S. and worldwide. The World Health Organization (WHO) estimates that 61 percent of all human diseases are zoonotic in origin, while 75 percent of new diseases discovered in the last decade are zoonotic.

Before the introduction of new hygiene regulations around 100 years ago, zoonotic diseases such as bovine tuberculosis, bubonic plague, and glanders caused millions of deaths. They are still a major problem in developing countries.

Causes

Zoonotic diseases can be transferred from animals to humans in several different ways.

Direct Contact

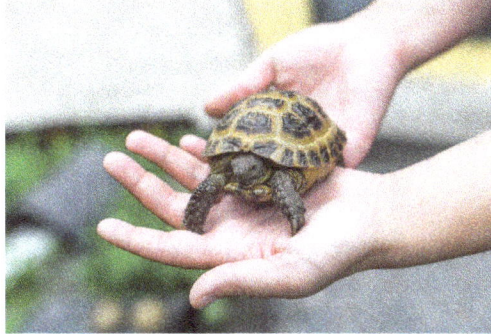

Direct contact is one potential cause of the spread of zoonotic diseases

Direct contact involves coming into contact with the bodily fluids of an infected animal, such as saliva, blood, urine, mucus, or feces.

This can happen because of merely touching or petting infected animals, or being bitten or scratched by one.

Water resources that are contaminated by manure can also contain a great variety of zoonotic bacteria and therefore increase the risk of that bacteria transferring to humans.

Indirect Contact

Indirect contact involves coming into contact with an area where infected animals live or roam, or by touching an object that has been contaminated by an infected animal.

Common areas where this occurs include:

- Aquarium tanks

- Chicken coops

- Pet baskets, cages, or kennels

- Pet food and water dishes

- Plants and soil where infected animals have been.

Farmers, abattoir workers, zoo or pet shop workers, and veterinarians have an increased risk of being exposed to zoonotic diseases. They can also become carriers and pass those diseases on to other people.

Vector-borne

A vector is a living organism that transfers an infection from an animal to a human, or another animal.

They are often arthropods. Common vectors include:

- Mosquitoes

- Ticks

- Fleas

- Lice.

The vector will bite the infected animal and then bite a human, passing on the zoonotic disease.

Food-borne

Zoonosis can come from contaminated animal food products, improper food handling, or inadequate cooking.

Around 1 in 6 American people will get sick at some point in their lives by eating or drinking contaminated food or drink.

Common causes of zoonosis through food-borne include:

- Unpasteurized milk

- Undercooked meat or eggs

- Raw fruit and vegetables contaminated with feces from an infected animal.

Other Causes

Global climate change, the overuse of antimicrobials in medicine, and more intensified farm settings are also thought to influence the increasing rate of zoonotic diseases.

People with a weakened immune system are also at greater risk. Common causes of immune-suppression include:

- Pregnancy

- Infancy

- Cancer treatment

- Organ transplant

- Diabetes

- Alcoholism

- Infectious diseases, such as AIDS.

Prevention

People come into contact with animals all the time, but there are several steps a person can take to help prevent infection. These include:

- Keeping hands clean: Washing hands with clean soap and running water after being around animals, even if not touching them, can stop germs spreading.

- Choosing a pet wisely: Thoroughly researching types of pets and taking steps to be safe around them can help prevent disease.

- Preventing bites from mosquitoes, ticks, and fleas: Using bug sprays, wearing long trousers and sleeves, and staying away from wooded areas can help prevent bites.

- Handling food safely: A person can prevent infections, such as salmonella, by ensuring food is cooked properly, that food preparation areas are clean, and by washing dishes and pots after use.

- Researching diseases before travel: Being aware of the different types of zoonotic diseases when traveling and taking precautionary steps with vaccines are essential.

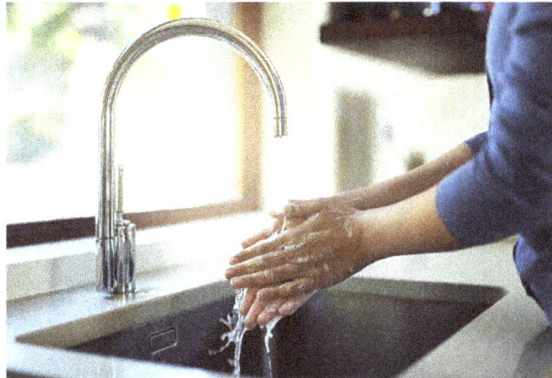

Practicing good hygiene by washing hands after handling animals and before preparing food may help to prevent the spread of zoonotic diseases

Anthrax

Anthrax is an infection caused by the bacterium *Bacillus anthracis*. It can occur in four forms: skin, lungs, intestinal, and injection. Symptoms begin between one day and two months after the infection is contracted. The skin form presents with a small blister with surrounding swelling that often turns into a painless ulcer with a black center. The inhalation form presents with fever, chest pain, and shortness of breath. The intestinal form presents with diarrhea which may contain blood, abdominal pains, and nausea and vomiting. The injection form presents with fever and an abscess at the site of drug injection.

Anthrax is spread by contact with the bacterium's spores, which often appear in infectious animal products. Contact is by breathing, eating, or through an area of broken skin. It does not typically spread directly between people. Risk factors include people who work with animals or animal products, travelers, postal workers, and military personnel. Diagnosis can be confirmed based on finding antibodies or the toxin in the blood or by culture of a sample from the infected site.

Anthrax vaccination is recommended for people who are at high risk of infection. Immunizing animals against anthrax is recommended in areas where previous infections have occurred. Two months of antibiotics such as ciprofloxacin, levofloxacin, and doxycycline after exposure can also prevent infection. If infection occurs treatment is with antibiotics and possibly antitoxin. The type and number of antibiotics used depends on the type of infection. Antitoxin is recommended for those with widespread infection.

Although a rare disease, human anthrax, when it does occur, is most common in Africa and central and southern Asia. It also occurs more regularly in Southern Europe than elsewhere on the continent, and is uncommon in Northern Europe and North America. Globally, at least 2,000 cases occur a year with about two cases a year in the United States. Skin infections represent more than 95% of cases. Without treatment, the risk of death from skin anthrax is 24%. For intestinal infection, the risk of death is 25 to 75%, while respiratory anthrax has a mortality of 50 to 80%, even with treatment. Until the 20th century, anthrax infections killed hundreds of thousands of people and animals each year. Anthrax has been developed as a weapon by a number of countries. In plant-eating animals, infection occurs when they eat or breathe in the spores while grazing. Carnivores may become infected by eating infected animals.

Signs and Symptoms

Skin

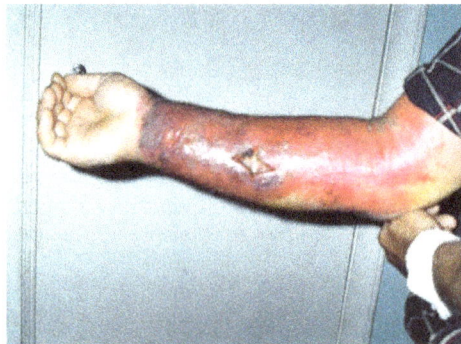

Skin lesion from anthrax

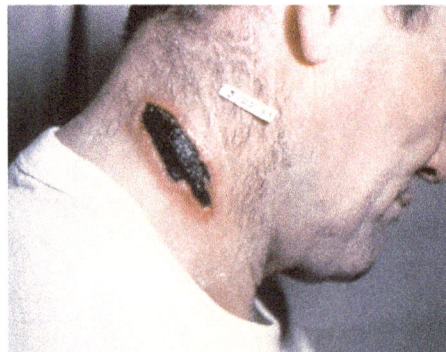

Skin anthrax lesion on the neck

Cutaneous anthrax, also known as hide-porter's disease, is when anthrax occurs on the skin. It is the most common form (>90% of anthrax cases). It is also the least dangerous form (low mortality with treatment, 20% mortality without). Cutaneous anthrax presents as a boil-like skin lesion that eventually forms an ulcer with a black center (eschar). The black eschar often shows up as a large, painless, necrotic ulcer (beginning as an irritating and itchy skin lesion or blister that is dark and usually concentrated as a black dot, somewhat resembling bread mold) at the site of infection. In general, cutaneous infections form within the site of spore penetration between two and five days after exposure. Unlike bruises or most other lesions, cutaneous anthrax infections normally do not cause pain. Nearby lymph nodes may become infected, reddened, swollen, and painful. A scab forms over the lesion soon, and falls off in a few weeks. Complete recovery may take longer. Cutaneous anthrax is typically caused when *B. anthracis* spores enter through cuts on the skin. This form is found most commonly when humans handle infected animals and animal products.

Cutaneous anthrax is rarely fatal if treated, because the infection area is limited to the skin, preventing the lethal factor, edema factor, and protective antigen from entering and destroying a vital organ. Without treatment, about 20% of cutaneous skin infection cases progress to toxemia and death.

Lungs

Respiratory infection in humans is relatively rare and presents as two stages. It infects the lymph nodes in the chest first, rather than the lungs themselves, a condition called hemorrhagic mediastinitis, causing bloody fluid to accumulate in the chest cavity, therefore causing shortness of breath. The first stage causes cold and flu-like symptoms. Symptoms include fever, shortness of breath, cough, fatigue, and chills. This can last hours to days. Often, many fatalities from inhalational anthrax are when the first stage is mistaken for the cold or flu and the victim does not seek treatment until the second stage, which is 90% fatal. The second (pneumonia) stage occurs when the infection spreads from the lymph nodes to the lungs. Symptoms of the second stage develop suddenly after hours or days of the first stage. Symptoms include high fever, extreme shortness of breath, shock, and rapid death within 48 hours in fatal cases. Historical mortality rates were over 85%, but when treated early), observed case fatality rate dropped to 45%. Distinguishing pulmonary anthrax from more common causes of respiratory illness is essential to avoiding delays in diagnosis and thereby improving outcomes. An algorithm for this purpose has been developed.

Gastrointestinal

Gastrointestinal (GI) infection is most often caused by consuming anthrax-infected meat and is characterized by diarrhea, potentially with blood, abdominal pains, acute inflammation of the intestinal tract, and loss of appetite. Occasional vomiting of blood can occur. Lesions have been found in the intestines and in the mouth and throat. After the bacterium invades the gastrointestinal system, it spreads to the bloodstream and throughout the body, while continuing to make toxins. GI infections can be treated, but usually result in fatality rates of 25% to 60%, depending upon how soon treatment commences. This form of anthrax is the rarest.

Cause

Bacteria

Bacillus anthracis is a rod-shaped, Gram-positive, facultative anaerobic bacterium about 1 by 9 μm in size. It was shown to cause disease by Robert Koch in 1876 when he took a blood sample from an infected cow, isolated the bacteria, and put them into a mouse. The bacterium normally rests in spore form in the soil, and can survive for decades in this state. Herbivores are often infected whilst grazing, especially when eating rough, irritant, or spiky vegetation; the vegetation has been hypothesized to cause wounds within the GI tract, permitting entry of the bacterial spores into the tissues, though this has not been proven. Once ingested or placed in an open wound, the bacteria begin multiplying inside the animal or human and typically kill the host within a few days or weeks. The spores germinate at the site of entry into the tissues and then spread by the circulation to the lymphatics, where the bacteria multiply.

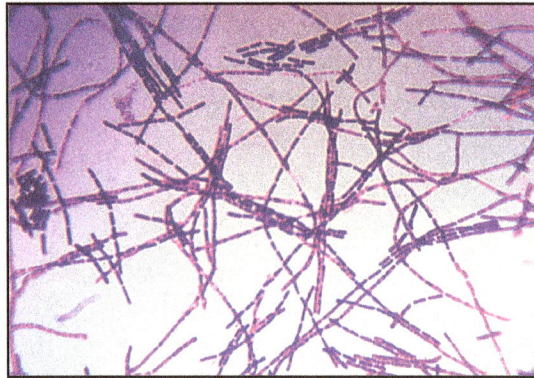

Photomicrograph of a Gram stain of the bacterium *Bacillus anthracis*, the cause of the anthrax disease

The production of two powerful exotoxins and lethal toxin by the bacteria causes death. Veterinarians can often tell a possible anthrax-induced death by its sudden occurrence, and by the dark, non-clotting blood that oozes from the body orifices. Most anthrax bacteria inside the body after death are outcompeted and destroyed by anaerobic bacteria within minutes to hours *post mortem*. However, anthrax vegetative bacteria that escape the body via oozing blood or through the opening of the carcass may form hardy spores. These vegetative bacteria are not contagious. One spore forms per one vegetative bacterium. The triggers for spore formation are not yet known, though oxygen tension and lack of nutrients may play roles. Once formed, these spores are very hard to eradicate.

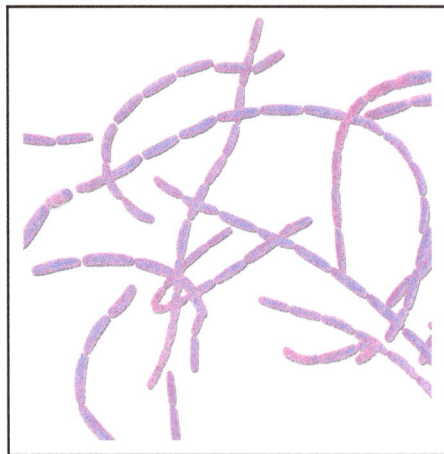

Bacillus anthracis

The infection of herbivores (and occasionally humans) by the inhalational route normally proceeds as: Once the spores are inhaled, they are transported through the air passages into the tiny air sacs (alveoli) in the lungs. The spores are then picked up by scavenger cells (macrophages) in the lungs and are transported through small vessels (lymphatics) to the lymph nodes in the central chest cavity (mediastinum). Damage caused by the anthrax spores and bacilli to the central chest cavity can cause chest pain and difficulty in breathing. Once in the lymph nodes, the spores germinate into active bacilli that multiply and eventually burst the macrophages, releasing many more bacilli into the bloodstream to be transferred to the entire body. Once in the blood stream, these bacilli release three proteins named lethal factor, edema factor, and protective antigen. The three are not toxic by themselves, but their combination is incredibly lethal to humans. Protective antigen combines with these other two factors to form lethal toxin and edema toxin, respectively. These toxins are the primary agents of tissue destruction, bleeding, and death of the host. If antibiotics are administered too late, even if the antibiotics eradicate the bacteria, some hosts still die of toxemia because the toxins produced by the bacilli remain in their systems at lethal dose levels.

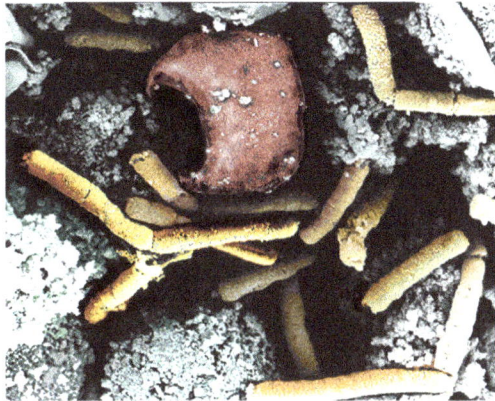

Color-enhanced scanning electron micrograph shows splenic tissue from a monkey with inhalational anthrax; featured are rod-shaped bacilli (yellow) and an erythrocyte (red)

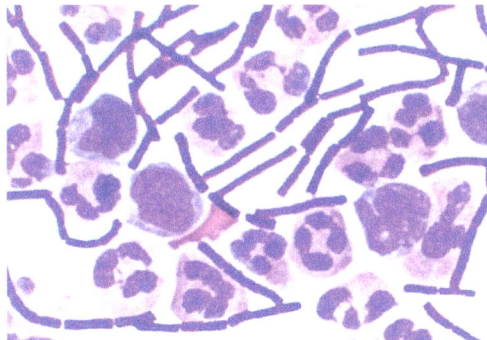

Gram-positive anthrax bacteria (purple rods) in cerebrospinal fluid: If present, a Gram negative bacterial species would appear pink

Exposure

The spores of anthrax are able to survive in harsh conditions for decades or even centuries. Such spores can be found on all continents, including Antarctica. Disturbed grave sites of infected animals have been known to cause infection after 70 years.

Occupational exposure to infected animals or their products (such as skin, wool, and meat) is the usual pathway of exposure for humans. Workers who are exposed to dead animals and animal products are at the highest risk, especially in countries where anthrax is more common. Anthrax in livestock grazing on open range where they mix with wild animals still occasionally occurs in the United States and elsewhere. Many workers who deal with wool and animal hides are routinely exposed to low levels of anthrax spores, but most exposure levels are not sufficient to develop anthrax infections. A lethal infection is reported to result from inhalation of about 10,000–20,000 spores, though this dose varies among host species. Little documented evidence is available to verify the exact or average number of spores needed for infection.

Historically, inhalational anthrax was called woolsorters' disease because it was an occupational hazard for people who sorted wool. Today, this form of infection is extremely rare in advanced nations, as almost no infected animals remain.

Mode of Infection

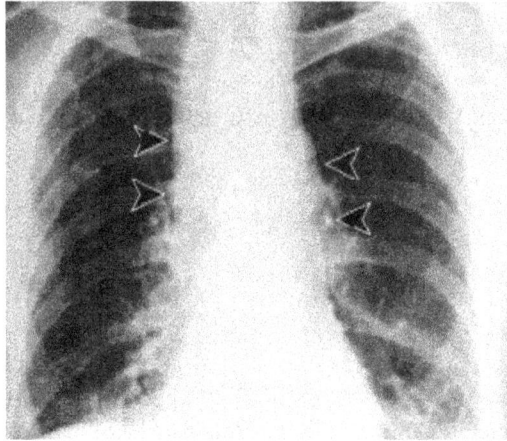

Inhalational anthrax, mediastinal widening

Anthrax can enter the human body through the intestines (ingestion), lungs (inhalation), or skin (cutaneous) and causes distinct clinical symptoms based on its site of entry. In general, an infected human is quarantined. However, anthrax does not usually spread from an infected human to an uninfected human. If the disease is fatal to the person's body, though, its mass of anthrax bacilli becomes a potential source of infection to others and special precautions should be used to prevent further contamination. Inhalational anthrax, if left untreated until obvious symptoms occur, is usually fatal.

Anthrax can be contracted in laboratory accidents or by handling infected animals, their wool, or their hides. It has also been used in biological warfare agents and by terrorists to intentionally infect as exemplified by the 2001 anthrax attacks.

Mechanism

The lethality of the anthrax disease is due to the bacterium's two principal virulence factors: the poly-D-glutamic acid capsule, which protects the bacterium from phagocytosis by host neutrophils, and the tripartite protein toxin, called anthrax toxin. Anthrax toxin is a mixture of three protein components: protective antigen (PA), edema factor (EF), and lethal factor (LF). PA plus LF produces lethal toxin, and PA plus EF produces edema toxin. These toxins cause death and tissue swelling (edema), respectively.

To enter the cells, the edema and lethal factors use another protein produced by *B. anthracis* called protective antigen, which binds to two surface receptors on the host cell. A cell protease then cleaves PA into two fragments: PA_{20} and PA_{63}. PA_{20} dissociates into the extracellular medium, playing no further role in the toxic cycle. PA_{63} then oligomerizes with six other PA_{63} fragments forming a heptameric ring-shaped structure named a prepore. Once in this shape, the complex can competitively bind up to three EFs or LFs, forming a resistant complex. Receptor-mediated endocytosis occurs next, providing the newly formed toxic complex access to the interior of the host cell. The acidified environment within the endosome triggers the heptamer to release the LF and/or EF into the cytosol. It is unknown how exactly the complex results in the death of the cell.

Edema factor is a calmodulin-dependent adenylate cyclase. Adenylate cyclase catalyzes the conversion of ATP into cyclic AMP (cAMP) and pyrophosphate. The complexation of adenylate cyclase with calmodulin removes calmodulin from stimulating calcium-triggered signaling, thus inhibiting the immune response. To be specific, LF inactivates neutrophils (a type of phagocytic cell) by the process just described so they cannot phagocytose bacteria. Throughout history, lethal factor was presumed to cause macrophages to make TNF-alpha and interleukin 1, beta (IL1B). TNF-alpha is a cytokine whose primary role is to regulate immune cells, as well as to induce inflammation and apoptosis or programmed cell death. Interleukin 1, beta is another cytokine that also regulates inflammation and apoptosis. The overproduction of TNF-alpha and IL1B ultimately leads to septic shock and death. However, recent evidence indicates anthrax also targets endothelial cells that line serous cavities such as the pericardial cavity, pleural cavity, and peritoneal cavity, lymph vessels, and blood vessels, causing vascular leakage of fluid and cells, and ultimately hypovolemic shock and septic shock.

Diagnosis

Various techniques may be used for the direct identification of *B. anthracis* in clinical material. Firstly, specimens may be Gram stained. *Bacillus* spp. are quite large in size (3 to 4 μm long), they may grow in long chains, and they stain Gram-positive. To confirm the organism is *B. anthracis*, rapid diagnostic techniques such as polymerase chain reaction-based assays and immunofluorescence microscopy may be used.

All *Bacillus* species grow well on 5% sheep blood agar and other routine culture media. Polymyxin-lysozyme-EDTA-thallous acetate can be used to isolate *B. anthracis* from contaminated specimens, and bicarbonate agar is used as an identification method to induce capsule formation. *Bacillus* spp. usually grow within 24 hours of incubation at 35 °C, in ambient air (room temperature) or in 5% CO_2. If bicarbonate agar is used for identification, then the medium must be incubated in 5% CO_2. *B. anthracis* colonies are medium-large, gray, flat, and irregular with swirling projections, often referred to as having a "medusa head" appearance, and are not hemolytic on 5% sheep blood agar. The bacteria are not motile, susceptible to penicillin, and produce a wide zone of lecithinase on egg yolk agar. Confirmatory testing to identify *B. anthracis* includes gamma bacteriophage testing, indirect hemagglutination, and enzyme-linked immunosorbent assay to detect antibodies. The best confirmatory precipitation test for anthrax is the Ascoli test.

Prevention

If a person is suspected as having died from anthrax, precautions should be taken to avoid skin contact with the potentially contaminated body and fluids exuded through natural body openings. The body should be put in strict quarantine. A blood sample should then be collected and sealed in a container and analyzed in an approved laboratory to ascertain if anthrax is the cause of death. Then, the body should be incinerated. Microscopic visualization of the encapsulated bacilli, usually in very large numbers, in a blood smear stained with polychrome methylene blue (McFadyean stain) is fully diagnostic, though culture of the organism is still the gold standard for diagnosis. Full isolation of the body is important to prevent possible contamination of others. Protective, impermeable clothing and equipment such as rubber gloves, rubber apron, and rubber boots with no perforations should be used when handling the body. No skin, especially if it has any wounds or scratches, should be exposed. Disposable personal protective equipment is preferable, but if not available, decontamination can be achieved by autoclaving. Disposable personal protective equipment and filters should be autoclaved, and/or burned and buried. Anyone working with anthrax in a suspected or confirmed person should wear respiratory equipment capable of filtering particles of their size or smaller. The US National Institute for Occupational Safety and Health – and Mine Safety and Health Administration-approved high-efficiency respirator, such as a half-face disposable respirator with a high-efficiency particulate air filter, is recommended. All possibly contaminated bedding or clothing should be isolated in double plastic bags and treated as possible biohazard waste. The body of an infected person should be sealed in an airtight body bag. Dead people who are opened and not burned provide an ideal source of anthrax spores. Cremating people is the preferred way of handling body disposal. No embalming or autopsy should be attempted without a fully equipped biohazard laboratory and trained, knowledgeable personnel.

Vaccines

Vaccines against anthrax for use in livestock and humans have had a prominent place in the history of medicine. The French scientist Louis Pasteur developed the first effective vaccine in 1881. Human anthrax vaccines were developed by the Soviet Union in the late 1930s and in the US and UK in the 1950s. The current FDA-approved US vaccine was formulated in the 1960s.

Currently administered human anthrax vaccines include acellular (United States) and live vaccine (Russia) varieties. All currently used anthrax vaccines show considerable local and general reactogenicity (erythema, induration, soreness, fever) and serious adverse reactions occur in about 1% of recipients. The American product, BioThrax, is licensed by the FDA and was formerly administered in a six-dose primary series at 0, 2, 4 weeks and 6, 12, 18 months, with annual boosters to maintain immunity. In 2008, the FDA approved omitting the week-2 dose, resulting in the currently recommended five-dose series. New second-generation vaccines currently being researched include recombinant live vaccines and recombinant subunit vaccines. In the 20th century the use of a modern product (BioThrax) to protect American troops against the use of anthrax in biological warfare was controversial.

Antibiotics

Preventive antibiotics are recommended in those who have been exposed. Early detection of sources of anthrax infection can allow preventive measures to be taken. In response to the anthrax attacks of October 2001, the United States Postal Service (USPS) installed biodetection systems (BDSs) in their large-scale mail processing facilities. BDS response plans were formulated by the USPS in conjunction with local responders including fire, police, hospitals, and public health. Employees of these facilities have been educated about anthrax, response actions, and prophylactic medication. Because of the time delay inherent in getting final verification that anthrax has been used, prophylactic antibiotic treatment of possibly exposed personnel must be started as soon as possible.

Treatment

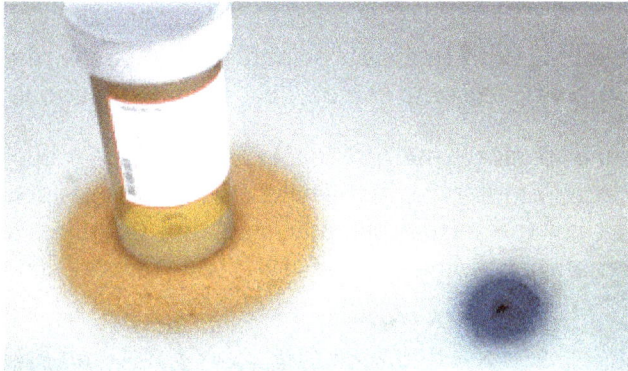

Anthrax and antibiotics

Anthrax cannot be spread directly from person to person, but a person's clothing and body may be contaminated with anthrax spores. Effective decontamination of people can be accomplished by a thorough wash-down with antimicrobial soap and water. Waste water should be treated with bleach or another antimicrobial agent. Effective decontamination of particles can be accomplished by boiling them in water for 30 minutes or longer. Chlorine bleach is ineffective in destroying spores and vegetative cells on surfaces, though formaldehyde is effective. Burning clothing is very effective in destroying spores. After decontamination, there is no need to immunize, treat, or isolate contacts of persons ill with anthrax unless they were also exposed to the same source of infection.

Antibiotics

Early antibiotic treatment of anthrax is essential; delay significantly lessens chances for survival. Treatment for anthrax infection and other bacterial infections includes large doses of intravenous and oral antibiotics, such as fluoroquinolones (ciprofloxacin), doxycycline, erythromycin, vancomycin, or penicillin. FDA-approved agents include ciprofloxacin, doxycycline, and penicillin.

In possible cases of pulmonary anthrax, early antibiotic prophylaxis treatment is crucial to prevent possible death.

In recent years, many attempts have been made to develop new drugs against anthrax, but existing drugs are effective if treatment is started soon enough.

Monoclonal Antibodies

In May 2009, Human Genome Sciences submitted a biologic license application (BLA, permission to market) for its new drug, raxibacumab (brand name ABthrax) intended for emergency treatment of inhaled anthrax. On 14 December 2012, the US Food and Drug Administration approved raxibacumab injection to treat inhalational anthrax. Raxibacumab is a monoclonal antibody that neutralizes toxins produced by *B. anthracis*. On March, 2016, FDA approved a second anthrax treatment using a monoclonal antibody which neutralizes the toxins produced by *B. anthracis*. Obiltoxaximab is approved to treat inhalational anthrax in conjunction with appropriate antibacterial drugs, and for prevention when alternative therapies are not available or appropriate.

Other Animals

Anthrax is especially rare in dogs and cats, as is evidenced by a single reported case in the United States in 2001. Anthrax outbreaks occur in some wild animal populations with some regularity.

Russian researchers estimate arctic permafrost contains around 1.5 million anthrax-infected reindeer carcasses, and the spores may survive in the permafrost for 105 years. A risk exists that global warming in the Arctic can thaw the permafrost, releasing anthrax spores in the carcasses. In 2016, an anthrax outbreak in reindeer was linked to a 75-year-old carcass that defrosted during a heat wave.

Ebola Virus Disease

Ebola virus disease (EVD), also known as Ebola hemorrhagic fever (EHF) or simply Ebola, is a viral hemorrhagic fever of humans and other primates caused by ebolaviruses. Signs and symptoms typically start between two days and three weeks after contracting the virus with a fever, sore throat, muscular pain, and headaches. Vomiting, diarrhea and rash usually follow, along with decreased function of the liver and kidneys. At this time, some people begin to bleed both internally and externally. The disease has a high risk of death, killing 25% to 90% of those infected, with an average of about 50%. This is often due to low blood pressure from fluid loss, and typically follows 6 to 16 days after symptoms appear.

The virus spreads through direct contact with body fluids, such as blood from infected humans or other animals. Spread may also occur from contact with items recently contaminated with bodily fluids. Spread of the disease through the air between primates, including humans, has not been documented in either laboratory or natural conditions. Semen or breast milk of a person after recovery from EVD may carry the virus for several weeks to months. Fruit bats are believed to be the normal carrier in nature, able to spread the virus without being affected by it. Other diseases such as malaria, cholera, typhoid fever, meningitis and other viral hemorrhagic fevers may resemble EVD. Blood samples are tested for viral RNA, viral antibodies or for the virus itself to confirm the diagnosis.

Control of outbreaks requires coordinated medical services and community engagement. This includes rapid detection, contact tracing of those who have been exposed, quick access to laboratory services, care for those infected, and proper disposal of the dead through cremation or burial. Samples of body fluids and tissues from people with the disease should be handled with special caution. Prevention includes limiting the spread of disease from infected animals to humans by handling potentially infected bushmeat only while wearing protective clothing, and by thoroughly cooking bushmeat before eating it. It also includes wearing proper protective clothing and washing hands when around a person with the disease. An Ebola vaccine has been studied in Africa with promising results. While there is no approved treatment for Ebola as of 2019, two treatments (REGN-EB3 and mAb114) are associated with improved outcomes. Supportive efforts, also, improve outcomes. This includes either oral rehydration therapy (drinking slightly sweetened and salty water) or giving intravenous fluids as well as treating symptoms.

The disease was first identified in 1976, in two simultaneous outbreaks: one in Nzara (a town in South Sudan) and the other in Yambuku (Democratic Republic of the Congo), a village near the Ebola River from which the disease takes its name. EVD outbreaks occur intermittently in tropical regions of sub-Saharan Africa. Between 1976 and 2013, the World Health Organization reports 24 outbreaks involving 2,387 cases with 1,590 deaths. The largest outbreak to date was the epidemic in West Africa, which occurred from December 2013, to January 2016, with 28,646 cases and 11,323 deaths. It was declared no longer an emergency on 29 March 2016. Other outbreaks in Africa began in the Democratic Republic of the Congo in May 2017, and 2018. In July 2019, the World Health Organization declared the Congo Ebola outbreak a world health emergency.

Signs and Symptoms

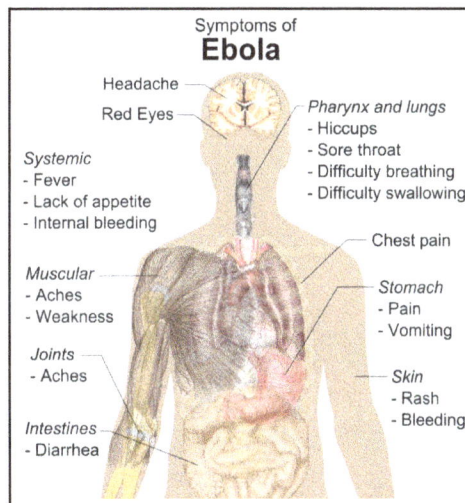

Signs and symptoms of Ebola

Onset

The length of time between exposure to the virus and the development of symptoms (incubation period) is between 2 and 21 days, and usually between 4 and 10 days. However, recent estimates based on mathematical models predict that around 5% of cases may take greater than 21 days to develop.

Symptoms usually begin with a sudden influenza-like stage characterized by feeling tired, fever, weakness, decreased appetite, muscular pain, joint pain, headache, and sore throat. The fever is usually higher than 38.3 °C (101 °F). This is often followed by nausea, vomiting, diarrhea, abdominal pain, and sometimes hiccups. The combination of severe vomiting and diarrhea often leads to severe dehydration. Next, shortness of breath and chest pain may occur, along with swelling, headaches, and confusion. In about half of the cases, the skin may develop a maculopapular rash, a flat red area covered with small bumps, five to seven days after symptoms begin.

Bleeding

In some cases, internal and external bleeding may occur. This typically begins five to seven days after the first symptoms. All infected people show some decreased blood clotting. Bleeding from mucous membranes or from sites of needle punctures has been reported in 40–50% of cases. This may cause vomiting blood, coughing up of blood, or blood in stool. Bleeding into the skin may create petechiae, purpura, ecchymoses or hematomas (especially around needle injection sites). Bleeding into the whites of the eyes may also occur. Heavy bleeding is uncommon; if it occurs, it is usually in the gastrointestinal tract. The incidence of bleeding into the gastrointestinal tract has decreased since earlier epidemics and is now estimated to be approximately 10% with improved prevention of disseminated intravascular coagulation.

Recovery and Death

Recovery may begin between 7 and 14 days after first symptoms. Death, if it occurs, follows typically 6 to 16 days from first symptoms and is often due to low blood pressure from fluid loss. In general, bleeding often indicates a worse outcome, and blood loss may result in death. People are often in a coma near the end of life.

Those who survive often have ongoing muscular and joint pain, liver inflammation, decreased hearing, and may have continued tiredness, continued weakness, decreased appetite, and difficulty returning to pre-illness weight. Problems with vision may develop.

Survivors develop antibodies against Ebola that last at least 10 years, but it is unclear whether they are immune to additional infections.

Cause

EVD in humans is caused by four of five viruses of the genus *Ebolavirus*. The four are Bundibugyo virus (BDBV), Sudan virus (SUDV), Taï Forest virus (TAFV) and one simply called Ebola virus (EBOV, formerly Zaire Ebola virus). EBOV, species *Zaire ebolavirus*, is the most dangerous of the known EVD-causing viruses, and is responsible for the largest number of outbreaks. The fifth virus, Reston virus (RESTV), is not thought to cause disease in humans, but has caused disease in other primates. All five viruses are closely related to marburgviruses.

Virology

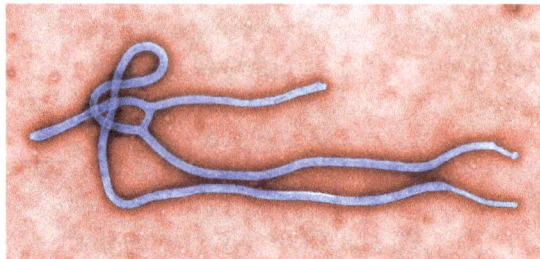

Electron micrograph of an Ebola virus virion

Ebolaviruses contain single-stranded, non-infectious RNA genomes. *Ebolavirus* genomes contain seven genes including 3'-UTR-*NP-VP35-VP40-GP-VP30-VP24-L*-5'-UTR. The genomes of the five different ebolaviruses (BDBV, EBOV, RESTV, SUDV and TAFV) differ in sequence and the number and location of gene overlaps. As with all filoviruses, ebolavirus virions are filamentous particles that may appear in the shape of a shepherd's crook, of a "U" or of a "6," and they may be coiled, toroid or branched. In general, ebolavirions are 80 nanometers (nm) in width and may be as long as 14,000 nm.

Their life cycle is thought to begin with a virion attaching to specific cell-surface receptors such as C-type lectins, DC-SIGN, or integrins, which is followed by fusion of the viral envelope with cellular membranes. The virions taken up by the cell then travel to acidic endosomes and lysosomes where the viral envelope glycoprotein GP is cleaved. This processing appears to allow the virus to bind to cellular proteins enabling it to fuse with internal cellular membranes and release the viral nucleocapsid. The *Ebolavirus* structural glycoprotein (known as GP1,2) is responsible for the virus' ability to bind to and infect targeted cells. The viral RNA polymerase, encoded by the *L* gene, partially uncoats the nucleocapsid and transcribes the genes into positive-strand mRNAs, which are then translated into structural and nonstructural proteins. The most abundant protein produced is the nucleoprotein, whose concentration in the host cell determines when L switches from gene transcription to genome replication. Replication of the viral genome results in full-length, positive-strand antigenomes that are, in turn, transcribed into genome copies of negative-strand virus progeny. Newly synthesized structural proteins and genomes self-assemble and accumulate near the inside of the cell membrane. Virions bud off from the cell, gaining their envelopes from the cellular membrane from which they bud. The mature progeny particles then infect other cells to repeat the cycle. The genetics of the Ebola virus are difficult to study because of EBOV's virulent characteristics.

Transmission

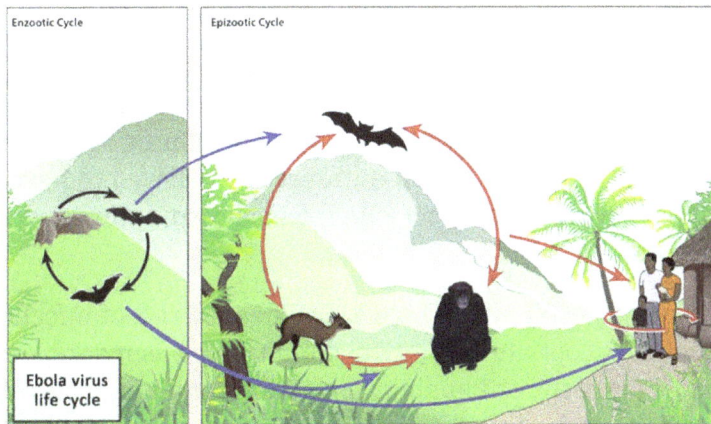

Life cycles of the *Ebolavirus*

It is believed that between people, Ebola disease spreads only by direct contact with the blood or other body fluids of a person who has developed symptoms of the disease. Body fluids that may contain Ebola viruses include saliva, mucus, vomit, feces, sweat, tears, breast milk, urine and semen. The WHO states that only people who are very sick are able to spread Ebola disease in saliva, and whole virus has not been reported to be transmitted through sweat. Most people spread the virus through blood, feces and vomit. Entry points for the virus include the nose, mouth, eyes, open wounds, cuts and abrasions. Ebola may be spread through large droplets; however, this is believed to occur only when a person is very sick. This contamination can happen if a person is splashed with droplets. Contact with surfaces or objects contaminated by the virus, particularly needles and syringes, may also transmit the infection. The virus is able to survive on objects for a few hours in a dried state, and can survive for a few days within body fluids outside of a person.

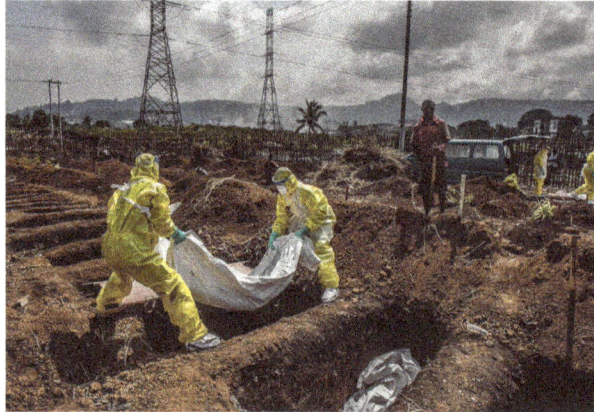
An illustration of safe burial practices

The Ebola virus may be able to persist for more than 3 months in the semen after recovery, which could lead to infections via sexual intercourse. Virus persistence in semen for over a year has been recorded in a national screening programme. Ebola may also occur in the breast milk of women after recovery, and it is not known when it is safe to breastfeed again. The virus was also found in the eye of one patient in 2014, two months after it was cleared from his blood. Otherwise, people who have recovered are not infectious.

The potential for widespread infections in countries with medical systems capable of observing correct medical isolation procedures is considered low. Usually when someone has symptoms of the disease, they are unable to travel without assistance.

Dead bodies remain infectious; thus, people handling human remains in practices such as traditional burial rituals or more modern processes such as embalming are at risk. 69% of the cases of Ebola infections in Guinea during the 2014 outbreak are believed to have been contracted via unprotected (or unsuitably protected) contact with infected corpses during certain Guinean burial rituals.

Health-care workers treating people with Ebola are at greatest risk of infection. The risk increases when they do not have appropriate protective clothing such as masks, gowns, gloves and eye protection; do not wear it properly; or handle contaminated clothing incorrectly. This risk is particularly common in parts of Africa where the disease mostly occurs and health systems function poorly. There has been transmission in hospitals in some African countries that reuse hypodermic needles. Some health-care centers caring for people with the disease do not have running water. In the United States the spread to two medical workers treating infected patients prompted criticism of inadequate training and procedures.

Human-to-human transmission of EBOV through the air has not been reported to occur during EVD outbreaks, and airborne transmission has only been demonstrated in very strict laboratory conditions, and then only from pigs to primates, but not from primates to primates. Spread of

EBOV by water, or food other than bushmeat, has not been observed. No spread by mosquitos or other insects has been reported. Other possible methods of transmission are being studied.

Airborne transmission among humans is theoretically possible due to the presence of Ebola virus particles in saliva, which can be discharged into the air with a cough or sneeze, but observational data from previous epidemics suggests the actual risk of airborne transmission is low. A number of studies examining airborne transmission broadly concluded that transmission from pigs to primates could happen without direct contact because, unlike humans and primates, pigs with EVD get very high ebolavirus concentrations in their lungs, and not their bloodstream. Therefore, pigs with EVD can spread the disease through droplets in the air or on the ground when they sneeze or cough. By contrast, humans and other primates accumulate the virus throughout their body and specifically in their blood, but not very much in their lungs. It is believed that this is the reason researchers have observed pig to primate transmission without physical contact, but no evidence has been found of primates being infected without actual contact, even in experiments where infected and uninfected primates shared the same air.

Initial Case

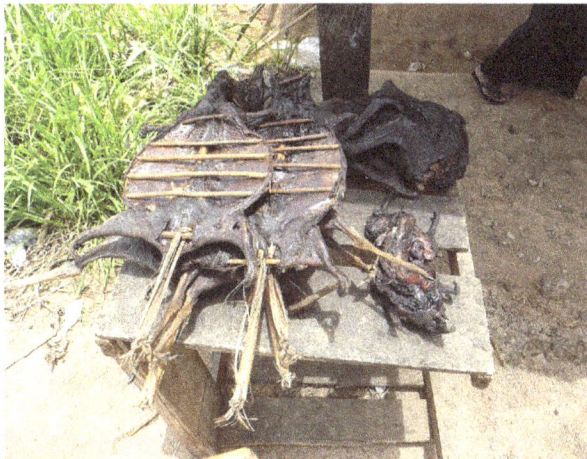

Bushmeat being prepared for cooking in Ghana. In Africa, wild animals including fruit bats are hunted for food and are referred to as bushmeat. In equatorial Africa, human consumption of bushmeat has been linked to animal-to-human transmission of diseases, including Ebola

Although it is not entirely clear how Ebola initially spreads from animals to humans, the spread is believed to involve direct contact with an infected wild animal or fruit bat. Besides bats, other wild animals sometimes infected with EBOV include several monkey species, chimpanzees, gorillas, baboons, and duikers.

Animals may become infected when they eat fruit partially eaten by bats carrying the virus. Fruit production, animal behavior and other factors may trigger outbreaks among animal populations.

Evidence indicates that both domestic dogs and pigs can also be infected with EBOV. Dogs do not appear to develop symptoms when they carry the virus, and pigs appear to be able to transmit the virus to at least some primates. Although some dogs in an area in which a human outbreak occurred had antibodies to EBOV, it is unclear whether they played a role in spreading the disease to people.

Reservoir

The natural reservoir for Ebola has yet to be confirmed; however, bats are considered to be the most likely candidate species. Three types of fruit bats (*Hypsignathus monstrosus*, *Epomops franqueti* and *Myonycteris torquata*) were found to possibly carry the virus without getting sick. As of 2013, whether other animals are involved in its spread is not known. Plants, arthropods, rodents, and birds have also been considered possible viral reservoirs.

Bats were known to roost in the cotton factory in which the first cases of the 1976 and 1979 outbreaks were observed, and they have also been implicated in Marburg virus infections in 1975 and 1980. Of 24 plant and 19 vertebrate species experimentally inoculated with EBOV, only bats became infected. The bats displayed no clinical signs of disease, which is considered evidence that these bats are a reservoir species of EBOV. In a 2002–2003 survey of 1,030 animals including 679 bats from Gabon and the Republic of the Congo, 13 fruit bats were found to contain EBOV RNA. Antibodies against Zaire and Reston viruses have been found in fruit bats in Bangladesh, suggesting that these bats are also potential hosts of the virus and that the filoviruses are present in Asia.

Between 1976 and 1998, in 30,000 mammals, birds, reptiles, amphibians and arthropods sampled from regions of EBOV outbreaks, no Ebola virus was detected apart from some genetic traces found in six rodents (belonging to the species *Mus setulosus* and *Praomys*) and one shrew (*Sylvisorex ollula*) collected from the Central African Republic. However, further research efforts have not confirmed rodents as a reservoir. Traces of EBOV were detected in the carcasses of gorillas and chimpanzees during outbreaks in 2001 and 2003, which later became the source of human infections. However, the high rates of death in these species resulting from EBOV infection make it unlikely that these species represent a natural reservoir for the virus.

Deforestation has been mentioned as a possible contributor to recent outbreaks, including the West African Ebola virus epidemic. Index cases of EVD have often been close to recently deforested lands.

Pathophysiology

Like other filoviruses, EBOV replicates very efficiently in many cells, producing large amounts of virus in monocytes, macrophages, dendritic cells and other cells including liver cells, fibroblasts, and adrenal gland cells. Viral replication triggers the high levels of inflammatory chemical signals and leads to a septic state.

EBOV is thought to infect humans through contact with mucous membranes or skin breaks. After infection, endothelial cells (cells lining the inside of blood vessels), liver cells, and several types of immune cells such as macrophages, monocytes, and dendritic cells are the main targets of attack. Following infection, immune cells carry the virus to nearby lymph nodes where further reproduction of the virus takes place. From there the virus can enter the bloodstream and lymphatic system and spread throughout the body. Macrophages are the first cells infected with the virus, and this infection results in programmed cell death. Other types of white blood cells, such as lymphocytes, also undergo programmed cell death leading to an abnormally low concentration of lymphocytes in the blood. This contributes to the weakened immune response seen in those infected with EBOV.

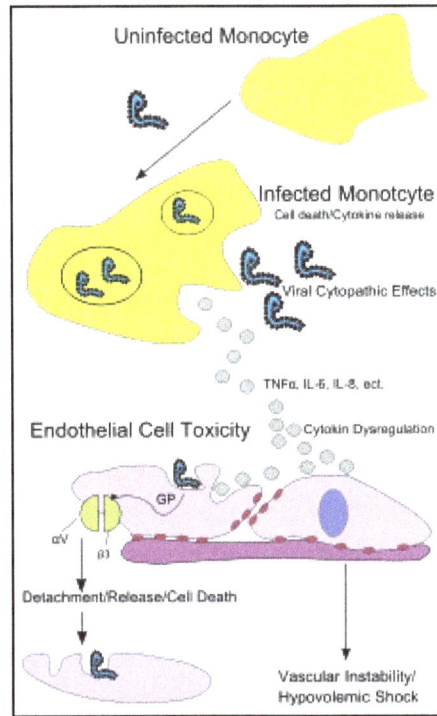

Pathogenesis schematic

Endothelial cells may be infected within three days after exposure to the virus. The breakdown of endothelial cells leading to blood vessel injury can be attributed to EBOV glycoproteins. This damage occurs due to the synthesis of Ebola virus glycoprotein (GP), which reduces the availability of specific integrins responsible for cell adhesion to the intercellular structure and causes liver damage, leading to improper clotting. The widespread bleeding that occurs in affected people causes swelling and shock due to loss of blood volume. The dysfunctional bleeding and clotting commonly seen in EVD has been attributed to increased activation of the extrinsic pathway of the coagulation cascade due to excessive tissue factor production by macrophages and monocytes.

After infection, a secreted glycoprotein, small soluble glycoprotein (sGP or GP) is synthesized. EBOV replication overwhelms protein synthesis of infected cells and the host immune defenses. The GP forms a trimeric complex, which tethers the virus to the endothelial cells. The sGP forms a dimeric protein that interferes with the signaling of neutrophils, another type of white blood cell. This enables the virus to evade the immune system by inhibiting early steps of neutrophil activation.

Immune System Evasion

Filoviral infection also interferes with proper functioning of the innate immune system. EBOV proteins blunt the human immune system's response to viral infections by interfering with the cells' ability to produce and respond to interferon proteins such as interferon-alpha, interferon-beta, and interferon gamma.

The VP24 and VP35 structural proteins of EBOV play a key role in this interference. When a cell is infected with EBOV, receptors located in the cell's cytosol (such as RIG-I and MDA5) or outside of the cytosol (such as Toll-like receptor 3 (TLR3), TLR7, TLR8 and TLR9) recognize infectious molecules associated with the virus. On TLR activation, proteins including interferon regulatory factor 3 and interferon regulatory factor 7 trigger a signaling cascade that leads to the expression of type 1 interferons. The type 1 interferons are then released and bind to the IFNAR1 and IFNAR2 receptors expressed on the surface of a neighboring cell. Once interferon has bound to its receptors on the neighboring cell, the signaling proteins STAT1 and STAT2 are activated and move to the cell's nucleus. This triggers the expression of interferon-stimulated genes, which code for proteins with antiviral properties. EBOV's V24 protein blocks the production of these antiviral proteins by preventing the STAT1 signaling protein in the neighboring cell from entering the nucleus. The VP35 protein directly inhibits the production of interferon-beta. By inhibiting these immune responses, EBOV may quickly spread throughout the body.

Diagnosis

When EVD is suspected, travel, work history, and exposure to wildlife are important factors with respect to further diagnostic efforts.

Laboratory Testing

Possible non-specific laboratory indicators of EVD include a low platelet count; an initially decreased white blood cell count followed by an increased white blood cell count; elevated levels of the liver enzymes alanine aminotransferase (ALT) and aspartate aminotransferase (AST); and abnormalities in blood clotting often consistent with disseminated intravascular coagulation (DIC) such as a prolonged prothrombin time, partial thromboplastin time, and bleeding time. Filovirions such as EBOV may be identified by their unique filamentous shapes in cell cultures examined with electron microscopy.

The specific diagnosis of EVD is confirmed by isolating the virus, detecting its RNA or proteins, or detecting antibodies against the virus in a person's blood. Isolating the virus by cell culture, detecting the viral RNA by polymerase chain reaction (PCR) and detecting proteins by enzyme-linked immunosorbent assay (ELISA) are methods best used in the early stages of the disease and also for detecting the virus in human remains. Detecting antibodies against the virus is most reliable in the later stages of the disease and in those who recover. IgM antibodies are detectable two days after symptom onset and IgG antibodies can be detected six to 18 days after symptom onset. During an outbreak, isolation of the virus with cell culture methods is often not feasible. In field or mobile hospitals, the most common and sensitive diagnostic methods are real-time PCR and ELISA. In 2014, with new mobile testing facilities deployed in parts of Liberia, test results were obtained 3–5 hours after sample submission. In 2015, a rapid antigen test which gives results in 15 minutes was approved for use by WHO. It is able to confirm Ebola in 92% of those affected and rule it out in 85% of those not affected.

Differential Diagnosis

Early symptoms of EVD may be similar to those of other diseases common in Africa, including malaria and dengue fever. The symptoms are also similar to those of other viral hemorrhagic fevers such as Marburg virus disease, Crimean Congo hemorrhagic fever, and Lassa fever.

The complete differential diagnosis is extensive and requires consideration of many other infectious diseases such as typhoid fever, shigellosis, rickettsial diseases, cholera, sepsis, borreliosis, EHEC enteritis, leptospirosis, scrub typhus, plague, Q fever, candidiasis, histoplasmosis, trypanosomiasis, visceral leishmaniasis, measles, and viral hepatitis among others.

Non-infectious diseases that may result in symptoms similar to those of EVD include acute promyelocytic leukemia, hemolytic uremic syndrome, snake envenomation, clotting factor deficiencies/platelet disorders, thrombotic thrombocytopenic purpura, hereditary hemorrhagic telangiectasia, Kawasaki disease, and warfarin poisoning.

Prevention

Vaccines

Many Ebola vaccine candidates had been developed in the decade prior to 2014, but as of November 2014, none had been approved for use in humans in the United States. In December 2016, Ebola was found to be 70–100% prevented by rVSV-ZEBOV vaccine, making it the first proven vaccine against the disease. More than 100,000 people have been vaccinated against Ebola as of 2019.

Infection Control

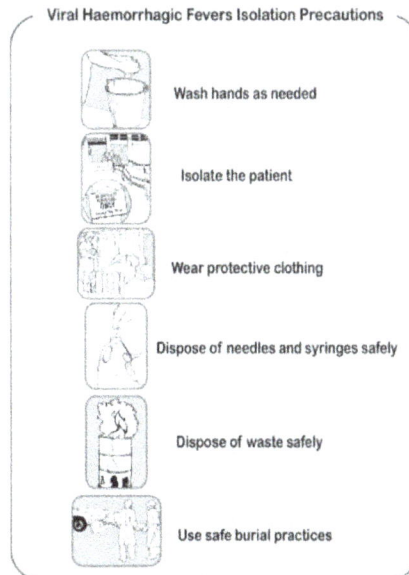

VHF isolation precautions poster

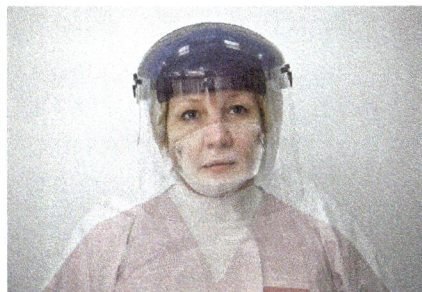

British woman wearing protective gear

People who care for those infected with Ebola should wear protective clothing including masks, gloves, gowns and goggles. The U.S. Centers for Disease Control (CDC) recommend that the protective gear leaves no skin exposed. These measures are also recommended for those who may handle objects contaminated by an infected person's body fluids. In 2014, the CDC began recommending that medical personnel receive training on the proper suit-up and removal of personal protective equipment (PPE); in addition, a designated person, appropriately trained in biosafety, should be watching each step of these procedures to ensure they are done correctly. In Sierra Leone, the typical training period for the use of such safety equipment lasts approximately 12 days.

The infected person should be in barrier-isolation from other people. All equipment, medical waste, patient waste and surfaces that may have come into contact with body fluids need to be disinfected. During the 2014 outbreak, kits were put together to help families treat Ebola disease in their homes, which included protective clothing as well as chlorine powder and other cleaning supplies. Education of caregivers in these techniques, and providing such barrier-separation supplies has been a priority of Doctors Without Borders.

Ebolaviruses can be eliminated with heat (heating for 30 to 60 minutes at 60 °C or boiling for 5 minutes). To disinfect surfaces, some lipid solvents such as some alcohol-based products, detergents, sodium hypochlorite (bleach) or calcium hypochlorite (bleaching powder), and other suitable disinfectants may be used at appropriate concentrations.

Education of the general public about the risk factors for Ebola infection and of the protective measures individuals may take to prevent infection is recommended by the World Health Organization. These measures include avoiding direct contact with infected people and regular hand washing using soap and water.

Bushmeat, an important source of protein in the diet of some Africans, should be handled and prepared with appropriate protective clothing and thoroughly cooked before consumption. Some research suggests that an outbreak of Ebola disease in the wild animals used for consumption may result in a corresponding human outbreak. Since 2003, such animal outbreaks have been monitored to predict and prevent Ebola outbreaks in humans.

If a person with Ebola disease dies, direct contact with the body should be avoided. Certain burial rituals, which may have included making various direct contacts with a dead body, require reformulation so that they consistently maintain a proper protective barrier between the dead body and the living. Social anthropologists may help find alternatives to traditional rules for burials.

Transportation crews are instructed to follow a certain isolation procedure, should anyone exhibit symptoms resembling EVD. As of August 2014, the WHO does not consider travel bans to be useful in decreasing spread of the disease. In October 2014, the CDC defined four risk levels used to determine the level of 21-day monitoring for symptoms and restrictions on public activities. In the United States, the CDC recommends that restrictions on public activity, including travel restrictions, are not required for the following defined risk levels:

- Having been in a country with widespread ebola disease transmission and having no known exposure (low risk); or having been in that country more than 21 days ago (no risk).

- Encounter with a person showing symptoms; but not within three feet of the person with ebola without wearing ppe; and no direct contact with body fluids.

- Having had brief skin contact with a person showing symptoms of ebola disease when the person was believed to be not very contagious (low risk).

- In countries without widespread ebola disease transmission; direct contact with a person showing symptoms of the disease while wearing ppe (low risk).

- Contact with a person with Ebola disease before the person was showing symptoms (no risk).

The CDC recommends monitoring for the symptoms of Ebola disease for those both at "low risk" and at higher risk.

In laboratories where diagnostic testing is carried out, biosafety level 4-equivalent containment is required. Laboratory researchers must be properly trained in BSL-4 practices and wear proper PPE.

Isolation

Isolation refers to separating those who are sick from those who are not. Quarantine refers to separating those who may have been exposed to a disease until they either show signs of the disease or are no longer at risk. Quarantine, also known as enforced isolation, is usually effective in decreasing spread. Governments often quarantine areas where the disease is occurring or individuals who may transmit the disease outside of an initial area. In the United States, the law allows quarantine of those infected with ebolaviruses.

Contact Tracing

Contact tracing is considered important to contain an outbreak. It involves finding everyone who had close contact with infected individuals and monitoring them for signs of illness for 21 days. If any of these contacts comes down with the disease, they should be isolated, tested and treated. Then the process is repeated, tracing the contacts' contacts.

Management

While there is no approved treatment for Ebola as of 2019, two treatments (REGN-EB3 and mAb114) are associated with improved outcomes. The Food and Drug Administration (FDA) advises people to be careful of advertisements making unverified or fraudulent claims of benefits supposedly gained from various anti-Ebola products.

Standard Support

Treatment is primarily supportive in nature. Early supportive care with rehydration and symptomatic treatment improves survival. Rehydration may be via the oral or intravenous route. These measures may include pain management, and treatment for nausea, fever, and anxiety. The World Health Organization (WHO) recommends avoiding aspirin or ibuprofen for pain management, due to the risk of bleeding associated with these medications.

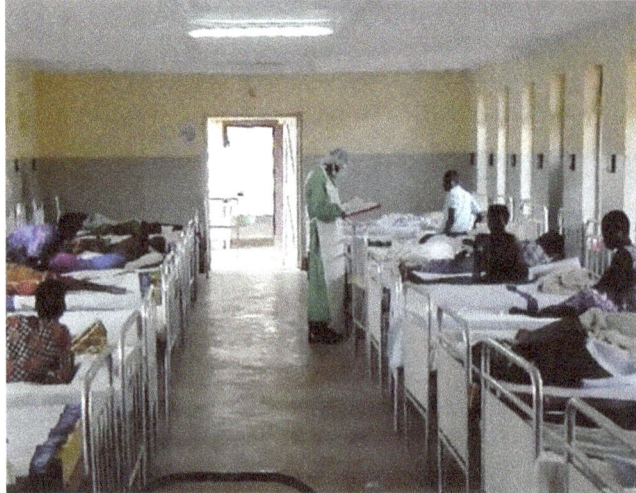

A hospital isolation ward

Blood products such as packed red blood cells, platelets, or fresh frozen plasma may also be used. Other regulators of coagulation have also been tried including heparin in an effort to prevent disseminated intravascular coagulation and clotting factors to decrease bleeding. Antimalarial medications and antibiotics are often used before the diagnosis is confirmed, though there is no evidence to suggest such treatment helps. Several experimental treatments are being studied.

Where hospital care is not possible, the WHO's guidelines for home care have been relatively successful. Recommendations include using towels soaked in a bleach solution when moving infected people or bodies and also applying bleach on stains. It is also recommended that the caregivers wash hands with bleach solutions and cover their mouth and nose with a cloth.

Intensive Care

Intensive care is often used in the developed world. This may include maintaining blood volume and electrolytes (salts) balance as well as treating any bacterial infections that may develop. Dialysis may be needed for kidney failure, and extracorporeal membrane oxygenation may be used for lung dysfunction.

Prognosis

EVD has a risk of death in those infected, between 25% and 90%. As of September 2014, the average risk of death among those infected is 50%. The highest risk of death was 90% in the 2002–2003 Republic of the Congo outbreak.

Death, if it occurs, follows typically six to sixteen days after symptoms appear and is often due to low blood pressure from fluid loss. Early supportive care to prevent dehydration may reduce the risk of death.

If an infected person survives, recovery may be quick and complete. Prolonged cases are often complicated by the occurrence of long-term problems, such as inflammation of the testicles, joint pains, fatigue, hearing loss, mood and sleep disturbances, muscular pain, abdominal pain, menstrual abnormalities, miscarriages, skin peeling, or hair loss. Inflammation and swelling of the uveal layer of the eye is the most common eye complication in survivors of Ebola virus disease. Eye symptoms, such as light sensitivity, excess tearing, and vision loss have been described.

Ebola can stay in some body parts like the eyes, breasts, and testicles after infection. Sexual transmission after recovery has been suspected. If sexual transmission occurs following recovery it is believed to be a rare event. One case of a condition similar to meningitis has been reported many months after recovery, as of October 2015.

A study of 44 survivors of the Ebola virus in Sierra Leone reported musculoskeletal pain in 70%, headache in 48%, and eye problems in 14%.

Other Animals

Wild Animals

Ebola has a high mortality rate among primates. Frequent outbreaks of Ebola may have resulted in the deaths of 5,000 gorillas. Outbreaks of Ebola may have been responsible for an 88% decline in tracking indices of observed chimpanzee populations in the 420 km^2 Lossi Sanctuary between 2002 and 2003. Transmission among chimpanzees through meat consumption constitutes a significant risk factor, whereas contact between the animals, such as touching dead bodies and grooming, is not.

Recovered gorilla carcasses have contained multiple Ebola virus strains, suggesting multiple introductions of the virus. Bodies decompose quickly and carcasses are not infectious after 3 to 4 days. Contact between gorilla groups is rare, suggesting that transmission among gorilla groups is unlikely, and that outbreaks result from transmission between viral reservoirs and animal populations.

Domestic Animals

In 2012, it was demonstrated that the virus can travel without contact from pigs to nonhuman primates, although the same study failed to achieve transmission in that manner between primates.

Dogs may become infected with EBOV but not develop symptoms. Dogs in some parts of Africa scavenge for food, and they sometimes eat EBOV-infected animals and also the corpses of humans. A 2005 survey of dogs during an EBOV outbreak found that although they remain asymptomatic, about 32 percent of dogs closest to an outbreak showed a seroprevalence for EBOV versus 9 percent of those farther away. The authors concluded that there were "potential implications for preventing and controlling human outbreaks."

Reston Virus

In late 1989, Hazelton Research Products' Reston Quarantine Unit in Reston, Virginia, suffered an outbreak of fatal illness amongst certain lab monkeys. This lab outbreak was initially diagnosed as simian hemorrhagic fever virus (SHFV) and occurred amongst a shipment of crab-eating macaque monkeys imported from the Philippines. Hazelton's veterinary pathologist sent tissue samples from dead animals to the United States Army Medical Research Institute of Infectious Diseases (USAMRIID) at Fort Detrick, Maryland, where an ELISA test indicated the antibodies present in the tissue were a response to Ebola virus and not SHFV. An electron microscopist from

USAMRIID discovered filoviruses similar in appearance to Ebola in the tissue samples sent from Hazelton Research Products' Reston Quarantine Unit.

A US Army team headquartered at USAMRIID euthanized the surviving monkeys, and brought all the monkeys to Ft. Detrick for study by the Army's veterinary pathologists and virologists, and eventual disposal under safe conditions. Blood samples were taken from 178 animal handlers during the incident. Of those, six animal handlers eventually seroconverted, including one who had cut himself with a bloody scalpel. Despite its status as a Level4 organism and its apparent pathogenicity in monkeys, when the handlers did not become ill, the CDC concluded that the virus had a very low pathogenicity to humans.

The Philippines and the United States had no previous cases of Ebola infection, and upon further isolation, researchers concluded it was another strain of Ebola, or a new filovirus of Asian origin, which they named *Reston ebolavirus* (RESTV) after the location of the incident. Reston virus (RESTV) can be transmitted to pigs. Since the initial outbreak it has since been found in nonhuman primates in Pennsylvania, Texas, and Italy, where the virus had infected pigs. According to the WHO, routine cleaning and disinfection of pig (or monkey) farms with sodium hypochlorite or detergents should be effective in inactivating the *Reston ebolavirus*. Pigs that have been infected with RESTV tend to show symptoms of the disease.

Cat-scratch Disease

Cat scratch disease	
Other names	Cat-scratch fever, Teeny's disease, inoculation lymphoreticulosis, subacute regional lymphadenitis
An enlarged lymph node in the armpit region of a person with cat-scratch disease, and wounds from a cat scratch on the hand.	
Specialty	Infectious disease
Symptoms	Bump at the site of the bite or scratch, swollen and painful lymph nodes
Complications	Encephalopathy, parotitis, endocarditis, hepatitis
Usual onset	Within 14 days after infection

Causes	Bartonella henselae from a cat bite or scratch
Diagnostic method	Based on symptoms, blood tests
Differential diagnosis	Adenitis, brucellosis, lymphogranuloma venereum, lymphoma, sarcoidosis
Treatment	Supportive treatment, antibiotics
Prognosis	Generally good, recovery within 4 months
Frequency	1 in 10,000 people

Cat-scratch disease (CSD) is an infectious disease that results from a scratch or bite of a cat. Symptoms typically include a non-painful bump or blister at the site of injury and painful and swollen lymph nodes. People may feel tired, have a headache, or a fever. Symptoms typically begin within 3-14 days following infection.

Cat-scratch disease is caused by the bacterium *Bartonella henselae* which is believed to be spread by the cat's saliva. Young cats pose a greater risk than older cats. Occasionally dog scratches or bites may be involved. Diagnosis is generally based on symptoms. Confirmation is possible by blood tests.

The primary treatment is supportive. Antibiotics speed healing and are recommended in those with severe disease or immune problems. Recovery typically occurs within 4 months but can require a year. About 1 in 10,000 people are affected. It is more common in children.

Signs and Symptoms

Cat-scratch disease commonly presents as tender, swollen lymph nodes near the site of the inoculating bite or scratch or on the neck, and is usually limited to one side. This condition is referred to as regional lymphadenopathy and occurs 1–3 weeks after inoculation. Lymphadenopathy in CSD most commonly occurs in the arms, neck, or jaw, but may also occur near the groin or around the ear. A vesicle or an erythematous papule may form at the site of initial infection. Most patients also develop systemic symptoms such as malaise, decreased appetite, and aches. Other associated complaints include headache, chills, muscular pains, joint pains, arthritis, backache, and abdominal pain. It may take 7 to 14 days, or as long as two months, for symptoms to appear. Most cases are benign and self-limiting, but lymphadenopathy may persist for several months after other symptoms disappear. The disease usually resolves spontaneously, with or without treatment, in one month.

In rare situations, CSD can lead to the development of serious neurologic or cardiac sequelae such as meningoencephalitis, encephalopathy, seizures, or endocarditis. Endocarditis associated with *Bartonella* infection has a particularly high mortality. Parinaud's oculoglandular syndrome is the most common ocular manifestation of CSD, and is a granulomatous conjunctivitis with concurrent swelling of the lymph node near the ear. Optic neuritis or neuroretinitis is one of the atypical presentations.

People who are immunocompromised are susceptible to other conditions associated with *B. henselae* and *B. quintana*, such as bacillary angiomatosis or bacillary peliosis. Bacillary angiomatosis is primarily a vascular skin lesion that may extend to bone or be present in other areas of the body. In the typical scenario, the patient has HIV or another cause of severe immune dysfunction. Bacillary peliosis is caused by *B. henselae* that most often affects patients with HIV and other conditions causing severe immune compromise. The liver and spleen are primarily affected, with findings of blood-filled cystic spaces on pathology.

Cause

Bartonella henselae is a fastidious, intracellular, Gram-negative bacterium.

Transmission

The cat was recognized as the natural reservoir of the disease in 1950 by Robert Debré. Kittens are more likely to carry the bacteria in their blood, so may be more likely to transmit the disease than adult cats. However, fleas serve as a vector for transmission of *B. henselae* among cats, and viable *B. henselae* are excreted in the feces of *Ctenocephalides felis*, the cat flea. Cats could be infected with *B. henselae* through intradermal inoculation using flea feces containing *B. henselae*. As a consequence, a likely means of transmission of *B. henselae* from cats to humans may be inoculation with flea feces containing *B. henselae* through a contaminated cat scratch wound or by cat saliva transmitted in a bite. Ticks can also act as vectors and occasionally transmit the bacteria to humans. Combined clinical and PCR-based research has shown that other organisms can transmit Bartonella, including spiders. Cryptic *Bartonella* infection may be a much larger problem than previously thought, constituting an unrecognized occupational health hazard of veterinarians.

Diagnosis

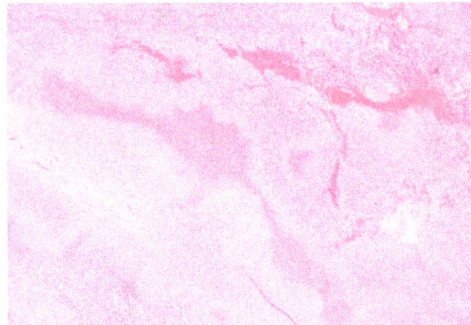

Micrograph of a lymph node affected by cat scratch disease. H&E stain

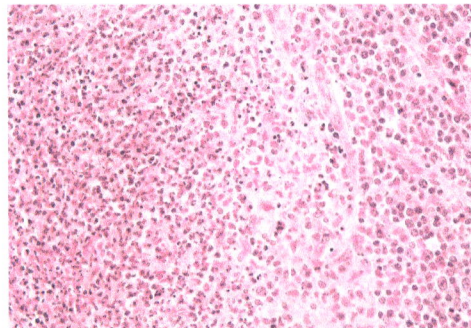

High-magnification micrograph of CSD showing a granuloma (pale cells - right of center on image) and a microabscess with neutrophils (left of image), H&E stain

The Warthin–Starry stain can be helpful to show the presence of *B. henselae*, but is often difficult to interpret. *B. henselae* is difficult to culture and can take 2–6 weeks to incubate. The best diagnostic method available is polymerase chain reaction, which has a sensitivity of 43-76% and a specificity (in one study) of 100%.

Histology

Cat-scratch disease is characterized by granulomatous inflammation on histological examination of the lymph nodes. Under the microscope, the skin lesion demonstrates a circumscribed focus of necrosis, surrounded by histiocytes, often accompanied by multinucleated giant cells, lymphocytes, and eosinophils. The regional lymph nodes demonstrate follicular hyperplasia with central stellate necrosis with neutrophils, surrounded by palisading histiocytes (suppurative granulomas) and sinuses packed with monocytoid B cells, usually without perifollicular and intrafollicular epithelioid cells. This pattern, although typical, is only present in a minority of cases.

Prevention

Cat-scratch disease can be primarily prevented by taking flea control measures and washing hands after handling a cat or cat feces; since cats are mostly exposed to fleas when they are outside, keeping cats inside can help prevent infestation.

Treatment

Most healthy people clear the infection without treatment, but in 5 to 14% of individuals, the organisms disseminate and infect the liver, spleen, eye, or central nervous system. Although some experts recommend not treating typical CSD in immunocompetent patients with mild to moderate illness, treatment of all patients with antimicrobial agents (Grade 2B) is suggested due to the probability of disseminated disease. The preferred antibiotic for treatment is azithromycin, since this agent is the only one studied in a randomized controlled study.

Azithromycin is preferentially used in pregnancy to avoid the teratogenic side effects of doxycycline. However, doxycycline is preferred to treat *B. henselae* infections with optic neuritis due to its ability to adequately penetrate the tissues of the eye and central nervous system.

Rat-bite Fever

Rat-bite fever is an acute, febrile human illness caused by bacteria transmitted by rodents, in most cases, which is passed from rodent to human by the rodent's urine or mucous secretions. Alternative names for rat-bite fever include streptobacillary fever, streptobacillosis, spirillary fever, bogger, and epidemic arthritic erythema. It is a rare disease spread by infected rodents and can be caused by two specific types of bacteria. Most cases occur in Japan, but specific strains of the disease are present in the United States, Europe, Australia, and Africa. Some cases are diagnosed after patients were exposed to the urine or bodily secretions of an infected animal. These secretions can come from the mouth, nose, or eyes of the rodent. The majority of cases are due to the animal's bite. It can also be transmitted through food or water contaminated with rat feces or urine. Other animals can be infected with this disease, including weasels, gerbils, and squirrels. Household pets such as dogs or cats exposed to these animals can also carry the disease and infect humans. If a person is bitten by a rodent, it is important to quickly wash and cleanse the wound area thoroughly with antiseptic solution to reduce the risk of infection.

Symptoms

Symptoms are different for every person depending on the type of rat-bite fever with which the person is infected. Both spirillary and streptobacillary rat-bite fever have a few individual symptoms, although most symptoms are shared. Streptobacillosis is most commonly found in the United States and spirillary rat-bite fever is generally diagnosed in patients in Africa. Rat-bite symptoms are visually seen in most cases and include inflammation around the open sore. A rash can also spread around the area and appear red or purple. Other symptoms associated with streptobacillary rat-bite fever include chills, fever, vomiting, headaches, and muscle aches. Joints can also become painfully swollen and pain can be experienced in the back. Skin irritations such as ulcers or inflammation can develop on the hands and feet. Wounds heal slowly, so symptoms possibly come and go over the course of a few months.

Symptoms associated with spirillary rat-bite fever include issues with the lymph nodes, which often swell or become inflamed as a reaction to the infection. The most common locations of lymph node swelling are in the neck, groin, and underarm. Symptoms generally appear within 2 to 10 days of exposure to the infected animal. It begins with the fever and progresses to the rash on the hands and feet within 2 to 4 days. Rash appears all over the body with this form, but rarely causes joint pain.

Causes

Two types of Gram-negative, facultatively anaerobic bacteria can cause the infection.

Spirillosis

Rat-bite fever transmitted by the Gram-negative coiled rod *Spirillum minus* (also known as *Spirillum minor*) is more rare, and is found most often in Asia. In Japan, the disease is called *sodoku*. Symptoms do not manifest for two to four weeks after exposure to the organism, and the wound through which it entered exhibits slow healing and marked inflammation. The fever lasts longer and is recurring, for months in some cases. Rectal pain and gastrointestinal symptoms are less severe or are absent. Penicillin is the most common treatment.

Streptobacillosis

The streptobacillosis form of rat-bite fever is known by the alternative names Haverhill fever and epidemic arthritic erythema. It is a severe disease caused by *Streptobacillus moniliformis*, transmitted either by rat bite or ingestion of contaminated products (Haverhill fever). After an incubation period of 2–10 days, Haverhill fever begins with high prostrating fevers, rigors (shivering), headache, and polyarthralgia (joint pain). Soon, an exanthem (widespread rash) appears, either maculopapular (flat red with bumps) or petechial (red or purple spots) and arthritis of large joints can be seen. The organism can be cultivated in blood or articular fluid. The disease can be fatal if untreated in 20% of cases due to malignant endocarditis, meningoencephalitis, or septic shock. Treatment is with penicillin, tetracycline, or doxycycline.

Diagnosis

This condition is diagnosed by detecting the bacteria in skin, blood, joint fluid, or lymph nodes. Blood antibody tests may also be used. To get a proper diagnosis for rat-bite fever, different tests are run depending on the symptoms being experienced.

To diagnosis streptobacillary rat-bite fever, blood or joint fluid is extracted and the organisms living in it are cultured. Diagnosis for spirillary rat bite fever is by direct visualization or culture of spirilla from blood smears or tissue from lesions or lymph nodes. Treatment with antibiotics is the same for both types of infection. The condition responds to penicillin, and where allergies to it occur, erythromycin or tetracyclines are used.

Prevention

While obviously preventable by staying away from rodents, otherwise hands and face should be washed after contact and any scratches both cleaned and antiseptics applied. The effect of chemoprophylaxis following rodent bites or scratches on the disease is unknown. No vaccines are available for these diseases. Improved conditions to minimize rodent contact with humans are the best preventive measures. Animal handlers, laboratory workers, and sanitation and sewer workers must take special precautions against exposure. Wild rodents, dead or alive, should not be touched and pets must not be allowed to ingest rodents. Those living in the inner cities where overcrowding and poor sanitation cause rodent problems are at risk from the disease. Half of all cases reported are children under 12 living in these conditions.

Prognosis

When proper treatment is provided for patients with rat-bite fever, the prognosis is positive. Without treatment, the infection usually resolves on its own, although it may take up to a year to do so. A particular strain of rat-bite fever in the United States can progress and cause serious complications that can be potentially fatal. Before antibiotics were used, many cases resulted in death. If left untreated, streptobacillary rat-bite fever can result in infection in the lining of the heart, covering over the spinal cord and brain, or in the lungs. Any tissue or organ throughout the body may develop an abscess.

Rabies

Rabies is a viral disease that causes inflammation of the brain in humans and other mammals. Early symptoms can include fever and tingling at the site of exposure. These symptoms are followed by one or more of the following symptoms: violent movements, uncontrolled excitement, fear of water, an inability to move parts of the body, confusion, and loss of consciousness. Once symptoms appear, the result is nearly always death. The time period between contracting the disease and the start of symptoms is usually one to three months, but can vary from less than one week to more than one year. The time depends on the distance the virus must travel along peripheral nerves to reach the central nervous system.

Rabies is caused by *lyssaviruses*, including the rabies virus and Australian bat lyssavirus. It is spread when an infected animal scratches or bites another animal or human. Saliva from an infected animal can also transmit rabies if the saliva comes into contact with the eyes, mouth, or nose. Globally, dogs are the most common animal involved. In countries where dogs commonly have the disease, more than 99% of rabies cases are the direct result of dog bites. In the Americas, bat bites are the most common source of rabies infections in humans, and less than 5% of cases are from dogs. Rodents are very rarely infected with rabies. The disease can be diagnosed only after the start of symptoms.

Animal control and vaccination programs have decreased the risk of rabies from dogs in a number of regions of the world. Immunizing people before they are exposed is recommended for those at high risk, including those who work with bats or who spend prolonged periods in areas of the world where rabies is common. In people who have been exposed to rabies, the rabies vaccine and sometimes rabies immunoglobulin are effective in preventing the disease if the person receives the treatment before the start of rabies symptoms. Washing bites and scratches for 15 minutes with soap and water, povidone-iodine, or detergent may reduce the number of viral particles and may be somewhat effective at preventing transmission. As of 2016, only fourteen people had survived a rabies infection after showing symptoms.

Rabies caused about 17,400 human deaths worldwide in 2015. More than 95% of human deaths from rabies occur in Africa and Asia. About 40% of deaths occur in children under the age of 15. Rabies is present in more than 150 countries and on all continents but Antarctica. More than 3 billion people live in regions of the world where rabies occurs. A number of countries, including Australia and Japan, as well as much of Western Europe, do not have rabies among dogs. Many Pacific islands do not have rabies at all. It is classified as a neglected tropical disease.

Signs and Symptoms

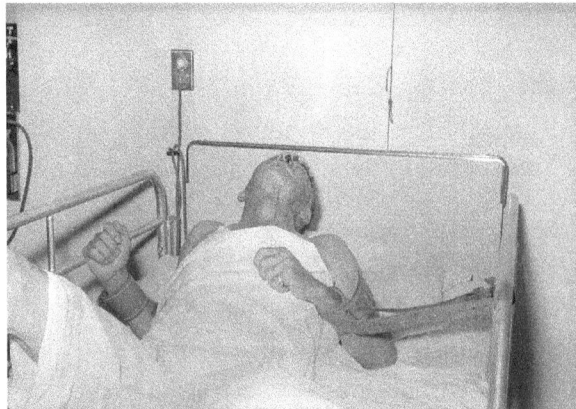

A man with rabies

The period between infection and the first symptoms (incubation period) is typically 1–3 months in humans. Incubation periods as short as four days and longer than six years have been documented, depending on the location and severity of the contaminated wound and the amount of virus introduced. Initial signs and symptoms of rabies are often nonspecific such as fever and headache. As rabies progresses and causes inflammation of the brain and/or meninges, signs and symptoms can include slight or partial paralysis, anxiety, insomnia, confusion, agitation, abnormal behavior, paranoia, terror, and hallucinations, progressing to delirium, and coma. The person may also have hydrophobia. Death usually occurs 2 to 10 days after first symptoms. Survival is almost unknown once symptoms have presented, even with the administration of proper and intensive care.

Fear of Water

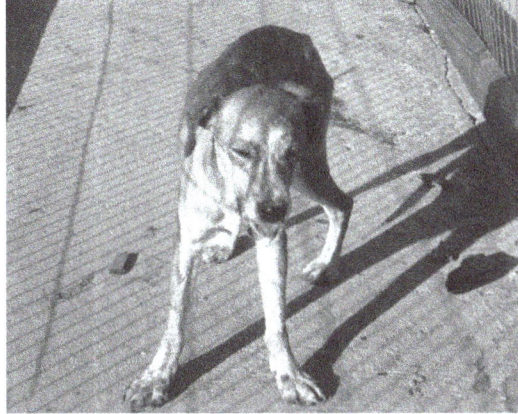
A rabid dog

Hydrophobia ("fear of water") is the historic name for rabies. It refers to a set of symptoms in the later stages of an infection in which the person has difficulty swallowing, shows panic when presented with liquids to drink, and cannot quench their thirst. Any mammal infected with the virus may demonstrate hydrophobia.

Saliva production is greatly increased, and attempts to drink, or even the intention or suggestion of drinking, may cause excruciatingly painful spasms of the muscles in the throat and larynx. This can be attributed to the fact that the virus multiplies and assimilates in the salivary glands of the infected animal with the effect of further transmission through biting. The ability to transmit the virus would decrease significantly if the infected individual could swallow saliva and water.

Hydrophobia is commonly associated with furious rabies, which affects 80% of rabies-infected people. The remaining 20% may experience a paralytic form of rabies that is marked by muscle weakness, loss of sensation, and paralysis; this form of rabies does not usually cause fear of water.

Cause

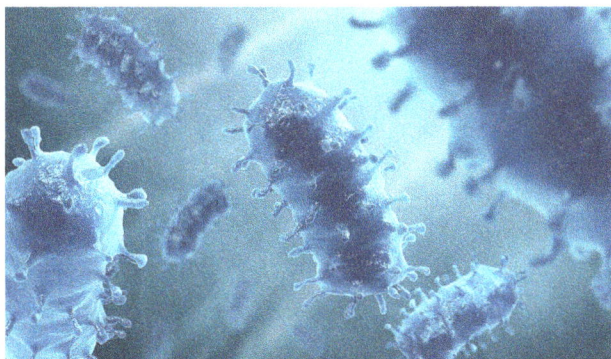
Drawing of the rabies virus

Rabies is caused by a number of *lyssaviruses* including the rabies virus and Australian bat lyssavirus.

The rabies virus is the type species of the *Lyssavirus* genus, in the family *Rhabdoviridae*, order *Mononegavirales*. Lyssavirions have helical symmetry, with a length of about 180 nm and a cross-section of about 75 nm. These virions are enveloped and have a single-stranded RNA genome with negative sense. The genetic information is packed as a ribonucleoprotein complex in which RNA is tightly bound by the viral nucleoprotein. The RNA genome of the virus encodes five genes whose order is highly conserved: nucleoprotein (N), phosphoprotein (P), matrix protein (M), glycoprotein (G), and the viral RNA polymerase (L).

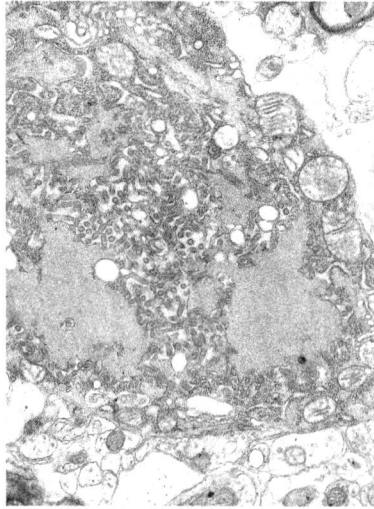

TEM micrograph with numerous rabies virions (small, dark grey, rodlike particles) and Negri bodies (the larger pathognomonic cellular inclusions of rabies infection)

Once within a muscle or nerve cell, the virus undergoes replication. The trimeric spikes on the exterior of the membrane of the virus interact with a specific cell receptor, the most likely one being the acetylcholine receptor. The cellular membrane pinches in a procession known as pinocytosis and allows entry of the virus into the cell by way of an endosome. The virus then uses the acidic environment, which is necessary, of that endosome and binds to its membrane simultaneously, releasing its five proteins and single strand RNA into the cytoplasm.

The L protein then transcribes five mRNA strands and a positive strand of RNA all from the original negative strand RNA using free nucleotides in the cytoplasm. These five mRNA strands are then translated into their corresponding proteins (P, L, N, G and M proteins) at free ribosomes in the cytoplasm. Some proteins require post-translative modifications. For example, the G protein travels through the rough endoplasmic reticulum, where it undergoes further folding, and is then transported to the Golgi apparatus, where a sugar group is added to it (glycosylation).

When there are enough viral proteins, the viral polymerase will begin to synthesize new negative strands of RNA from the template of the positive strand RNA. These negative strands will then form complexes with the N, P, L and M proteins and then travel to the inner membrane of the cell, where a G protein has embedded itself in the membrane. The G protein then coils around the N-P-L-M complex of proteins taking some of the host cell membrane with it, which will form the new outer envelope of the virus particle. The virus then buds from the cell.

From the point of entry, the virus is neurotropic, traveling along the neural pathways into the central nervous system. The virus usually first infects muscle cells close to the site of infection, where they are able to replicate without being 'noticed' by the host's immune system. Once enough virus has been replicated, they begin to bind to acetylcholine receptors at the neuromuscular junction. The virus then travels through the nerve cell axon via retrograde transport, as its P protein interacts with dynein, a protein present in the cytoplasm of nerve cells. Once the virus reaches the cell body it travels rapidly to the central nervous system (CNS), replicating in motor neurons and eventually reaching the brain. After the brain is infected, the virus travels centrifugally to the peripheral and autonomic nervous systems, eventually migrating to the salivary glands, where it is ready to be transmitted to the next host.

Transmission

All warm-blooded species, including humans, may become infected with the rabies virus and develop symptoms. Birds were first artificially infected with rabies in 1884; however, infected birds are largely, if not wholly, asymptomatic, and recover. Other bird species have been known to develop rabies antibodies, a sign of infection, after feeding on rabies-infected mammals.

The virus has also adapted to grow in cells of cold-blooded vertebrates. Most animals can be infected by the virus and can transmit the disease to humans. Infected bats, monkeys, raccoons, foxes, skunks, cattle, wolves, coyotes, dogs, cats, and mongooses (normally either the small Asian mongoose or the yellow mongoose) present the greatest risk to humans.

Rabies may also spread through exposure to infected bears, domestic farm animals, groundhogs, weasels, and other wild carnivorans. However, lagomorphs, such as hares and rabbits, and small rodents such as chipmunks, gerbils, guinea pigs, hamsters, mice, rats, and squirrels, are almost never found to be infected with rabies and are not known to transmit rabies to humans. Bites from mice, rats, or squirrels rarely require rabies prevention because these rodents are typically killed by any encounter with a larger, rabid animal, and would, therefore, not be carriers. The Virginia opossum is resistant but not immune to rabies.

The virus is usually present in the nerves and saliva of a symptomatic rabid animal. The route of infection is usually, but not always, by a bite. In many cases, the infected animal is exceptionally aggressive, may attack without provocation, and exhibits otherwise uncharacteristic behavior. This is an example of a viral pathogen modifying the behavior of its host to facilitate its transmission to other hosts.

Transmission between humans is extremely rare. A few cases have been recorded through transplant surgery. The only well-documented cases of rabies caused by human-to-human transmission occurred among eight recipients of transplanted corneas and among three recipients of solid organs. In addition to transmission from cornea and organ transplants, bite and non-bite exposures inflicted by infected humans could theoretically transmit rabies, but no such cases have been documented, since infected humans are usually hospitalized and necessary precautions taken. Casual contact, such as touching a person with rabies or contact with non-infectious fluid or tissue (urine, blood, feces) does not constitute an exposure and does not require post-exposure prophylaxis. Additionally, as the virus is present in sperm or vaginal secretions, spread through sex may be possible.

After a typical human infection by bite, the virus enters the peripheral nervous system. It then travels along the afferent nerves toward the central nervous system. During this phase, the virus cannot be easily detected within the host, and vaccination may still confer cell-mediated immunity to prevent symptomatic rabies. When the virus reaches the brain, it rapidly causes encephalitis, the prodromal phase, which is the beginning of the symptoms. Once the patient becomes symptomatic, treatment is almost never effective and mortality is over 99%. Rabies may also inflame the spinal cord, producing transverse myelitis.

Diagnosis

Rabies can be difficult to diagnose, because, in the early stages, it is easily confused with other diseases or with aggressiveness. The reference method for diagnosing rabies is the fluorescent antibody test (FAT), an immunohistochemistry procedure, which is recommended by the World Health Organization (WHO). The FAT relies on the ability of a detector molecule (usually fluorescein isothiocyanate) coupled with a rabies-specific antibody, forming a conjugate, to bind to and allow the visualisation of rabies antigen using fluorescent microscopy techniques. Microscopic analysis of samples is the only direct method that allows for the identification of rabies virus-specific antigen in a short time and at a reduced cost, irrespective of geographical origin and status of the host. It has to be regarded as the first step in diagnostic procedures for all laboratories. Autolysed samples can, however, reduce the sensitivity and specificity of the FAT. The RT PCR assays proved to be a sensitive and specific tool for routine diagnostic purposes, particularly in decomposed samples or archival specimens. The diagnosis can be reliably made from brain samples taken after death. The diagnosis can also be made from saliva, urine, and cerebrospinal fluid samples, but this is not as sensitive or reliable as brain samples. Cerebral inclusion bodies called Negri bodies are 100% diagnostic for rabies infection but are found in only about 80% of cases. If possible, the animal from which the bite was received should also be examined for rabies.

Some light microscopy techniques may also be used to diagnose rabies at a tenth of the cost of traditional fluorescence microscopy techniques, allowing identification of the disease in less-developed countries. A test for rabies, known as LN34, is easier to run on a dead animal's brain and might help determine who does and does not need post-exposure prevention. The test was developed by the CDC in 2018.

Differential Diagnosis

The differential diagnosis in a case of suspected human rabies may initially include any cause of encephalitis, in particular infection with viruses such as herpesviruses, enteroviruses, and arboviruses such as West Nile virus. The most important viruses to rule out are herpes simplex virus type one, varicella zoster virus, and (less commonly) enteroviruses, including coxsackieviruses, echoviruses, polioviruses, and human enteroviruses 68 to 71.

New causes of viral encephalitis are also possible, as was evidenced by the 1999 outbreak in Malaysia of 300 cases of encephalitis with a mortality rate of 40% caused by Nipah virus, a newly recognized paramyxovirus. Likewise, well-known viruses may be introduced into new locales, as is illustrated by the outbreak of encephalitis due to West Nile virus in the eastern United States. Epidemiologic factors, such as season, geographic location, and the patient's age, travel history, and possible exposure to bites, rodents, and ticks, may help direct the diagnosis.

Prevention

Almost all human cases of rabies were fatal until a vaccine was developed in 1885 by Louis Pasteur and Émile Roux. Their original vaccine was harvested from infected rabbits, from which the virus in the nerve tissue was weakened by allowing it to dry for five to ten days. Similar nerve tissue-derived vaccines are still used in some countries, as they are much cheaper than modern cell culture vaccines.

The human diploid cell rabies vaccine was started in 1967. Less expensive purified chicken embryo cell vaccine and purified vero cell rabies vaccine are now available. A recombinant vaccine called V-RG has been used in Belgium, France, Germany, and the United States to prevent outbreaks of rabies in undomesticated animals. Immunization before exposure has been used in both human and nonhuman populations, where, as in many jurisdictions, domesticated animals are required to be vaccinated.

The Missouri Department of Health and Senior Services Communicable Disease Surveillance 2007 Annual Report states the following can help reduce the risk of contracting rabies:

- Vaccinating dogs, cats, and ferrets against rabies.

- Keeping pets under supervision.

- Not handling wild animals or strays.

- Contacting an animal control officer upon observing a wild animal or a stray, especially if the animal is acting strangely.

- If bitten by an animal, washing the wound with soap and water for 10 to 15 minutes and contacting a healthcare provider to determine if post-exposure prophylaxis is required.

28 September is World Rabies Day, which promotes the information, prevention, and elimination of the disease.

Vaccinating other Animals

In Asia and in parts of the Americas and Africa, dogs remain the principal host. Mandatory vaccination of animals is less effective in rural areas. Especially in developing countries, pets may not be privately kept and their destruction may be unacceptable. Oral vaccines can be safely distributed in baits, a practice that has successfully reduced rabies in rural areas of Canada, France, and the United States. In Montreal, Quebec, Canada, baits are successfully used on raccoons in the Mount-Royal Park area. Vaccination campaigns may be expensive, and cost-benefit analysis suggests baits may be a cost-effective method of control. In Ontario, a dramatic drop in rabies was recorded when an aerial bait-vaccination campaign was launched.

The number of recorded human deaths from rabies in the United States has dropped from 100 or more annually in the early 20th century to one or two per year due to widespread vaccination of domestic dogs and cats and the development of human vaccines and immunoglobulin treatments. Most deaths now result from bat bites, which may go unnoticed by the victim and hence untreated.

Treatment

Treatment after exposure can prevent the disease if administered promptly, generally within 10 days of infection. Thoroughly washing the wound as soon as possible with soap and water for approximately five minutes is effective in reducing the number of viral particles. Povidone-iodine or alcohol is then recommended to reduce the virus further.

In the US, the Centers for Disease Control and Prevention recommends people receive one dose of human rabies immunoglobulin (HRIG) and four doses of rabies vaccine over a 14-day period. The immunoglobulin dose should not exceed 20 units per kilogram body weight. HRIG is expensive and constitutes most of the cost of post exposure treatment, ranging as high as several thousand dollars. As much as possible of this dose should be injected around the bites, with the remainder being given by deep intramuscular injection at a site distant from the vaccination site.

The first dose of rabies vaccine is given as soon as possible after exposure, with additional doses on days 3, 7 and 14 after the first. Patients who have previously received pre-exposure vaccination do not receive the immunoglobulin, only the postexposure vaccinations on days 0 and 3.

The pain and side effects of modern cell-based vaccines are similar to flu shots. The old nerve-tissue-based vaccinations that require multiple painful injections into the abdomen with a large needle are inexpensive, but are being phased out and replaced by affordable World Health Organization intradermal-vaccination regimens.

Intramuscular vaccination should be given into the deltoid, not the gluteal area, which has been associated with vaccination failure due to injection into fat rather than muscle. In infants, the lateral thigh is recommended.

Awakening to find a bat in the room, or finding a bat in the room of a previously unattended child or mentally disabled or intoxicated person, is an indication for post-exposure prophylaxis (PEP). The recommendation for the precautionary use of PEP in bat encounters where no contact is recognized has been questioned in the medical literature, based on a cost–benefit analysis. However, a 2002 study has supported the protocol of precautionary administering of PEP where a child or mentally compromised individual has been alone with a bat, especially in sleep areas, where a bite or exposure may occur with the victim being unaware. Begun with little or no delay, PEP is 100% effective against rabies. In the case in which there has been a significant delay in administering PEP, the treatment should be administered regardless, as it may still be effective. Every year, more than 15 million people get vaccination after potential exposure. While this works well, the cost is significant.

Milwaukee Protocol

The Milwaukee protocol, sometimes referred to as the Wisconsin protocol, is a method of attempted treatment of rabies infection in a human being. The treatment involves putting the person into a chemically induced coma and giving antiviral drugs. Jeanna Giese, who in 2004 was the first patient treated with the Milwaukee protocol, became the first person ever recorded to have survived rabies without receiving successful post-exposure prophylaxis. An intention-to-treat analysis has since found this protocol has a survival rate of about 8%. The protocol is not an effective treatment for rabies and its use is not recommended.

Prognosis

In unvaccinated humans, rabies is almost always fatal after neurological symptoms have developed.

Vaccination after exposure, PEP, is highly successful in preventing the disease if administered promptly, in general within six days of infection. Begun with little or no delay, PEP is 100% effective against rabies. In the case of significant delay in administering PEP, the treatment still has a chance of success.[

Toxocariasis

Toxocariasis is an illness of humans caused by larvae (immature worms) of either the dog roundworm (*Toxocara canis*), the cat roundworm (*Toxocara cati*) or the fox roundworm (*Toxocara canis*). Toxocariasis is often called visceral larva migrans (VLM). Depending on geographic location, degree of eosinophilia, eye and/or pulmonary signs, the terms ocular larva migrans (OLM), Weingarten's disease, Frimodt-Møller's syndrome, and eosinophilic pseudoleukemia are applied to toxocariasis. Other terms sometimes or rarely used include nematode ophthalmitis, toxocaral disease, toxocarose, and covert toxocariasis. This zoonotic, helminthic infection is a rare cause of blindness and may provoke rheumatic, neurologic, or asthmatic symptoms. Humans normally become infected by ingestion of embryonated eggs (each containing a fully developed second stage larva, L2) from contaminated sources (soil, undercooked meat, fresh or unwashed vegetables.)

Toxocara canis and *Toxocara cati* are perhaps the most ubiquitous gastrointestinal worms (helminths) of domestic dogs, cats, and foxes. There are many 'accidental' or paratenic hosts including humans, birds, pigs, rodents, goats, monkeys, and rabbits. In paratenic hosts, the larvae never mature and remain at the L2 stage.

There are three main syndromes: *visceral larva migrans* (VLM), which encompasses diseases associated with major organs; *covert toxocariasis*, which is a milder version of VLM; and *ocular larva migrans* (OLM), in which pathological effects on the host are restricted to the eye and the optic nerve.

Signs and Symptoms

Physiological reactions to *Toxocara* infection depend on the host's immune response and the parasitic load. Most cases of *Toxocara* infection are asymptomatic, especially in adults. When symptoms do occur, they are the result of migration of second stage *Toxocara* larvae through the body.

Covert toxocariasis is the least serious of the three syndromes and is believed to be due to chronic exposure. Signs and symptoms of covert toxocariasis are coughing, fever, abdominal pain, headaches, and changes in behavior and ability to sleep. Upon medical examination, wheezing, hepatomegaly, and lymphadenitis are often noted.

High parasitic loads or repeated infection can lead to visceral larva migrans (VLM). VLM is primarily diagnosed in young children, because they are more prone to exposure and ingestion of infective eggs. *Toxocara* infection commonly resolves itself within weeks, but chronic eosinophilia may result. In VLM, larvae migration incites inflammation of internal organs and sometimes the central nervous system. Symptoms depend on the organ(s) affected. Patients can present with pallor, fatigue, weight loss, anorexia, fever, headache, skin rash, cough, asthma, chest tightness, increased irritability, abdominal pain, nausea, and vomiting. Sometimes the subcutaneous migration tracks of the larvae can be seen. Patients are commonly diagnosed with pneumonia, bronchospasms, chronic pulmonary inflammation, hypereosinophilia, hepatomegaly, hypergammaglobulinaemia (IgM, IgG, and IgE classes), leukocytosis, and elevated anti-A and −B isohaemagglutinins. Severe cases have occurred in people who are hypersensitive to allergens; in rare cases, epilepsy, inflammation of the heart, pleural effusion, respiratory failure, and death have resulted from VLM.

Ocular larva migrans (OLM) is rare compared with VLM. A light *Toxocara* burden is thought to induce a low immune response, allowing a larva to enter the host's eye. Although there have been cases of concurrent OLM and VLM, these are extremely exceptional. OLM often occurs in just one eye and from a single larva migrating into and encysting within the orbit. Loss of vision occurs over days or weeks. Other signs and symptoms are red eye, white pupil, fixed pupil, retinal fibrosis, retinal detachment, inflammation of the eye tissues, retinal granulomas, and strabismus. Ocular granulomas resulting from OLM are frequently misdiagnosed as retinoblastomas. *Toxocara* damage in the eye is permanent and can result in blindness.

A case study published in 2008 supported the hypothesis that eosinophilic cellulitis may also be caused by infection with *Toxocara*. In this study, the adult patient presented with eosinophilic cellulitis, hepatosplenomegaly, anemia, and a positive ELISA for *T. canis*.

Incubation Period

The incubation period for *Toxocara canis* and *cati* eggs depends on temperature and humidity. *T. canis* females, specifically, are capable of producing up to 200,000 eggs a day that require 2–6 weeks minimum up to a couple months before full development into the infectious stage. Under ideal summer conditions, eggs can mature to the infective stage after two weeks outside of a host. Provided sufficient oxygen and moisture availability, *Toxocara* eggs can remain infectious for years, as their resistant outer shell enables the protection from most environmental threats. However, as identified in a case study presented within the journal of helminthology, the second stage of larvae development poses strict vulnerabilities to certain environmental elements. High temperatures and low moisture levels will quickly degrade the larvae during this stage of growth.

Toxocariasis	
Scientific classification	
Kingdom:	Animalia
Phylum:	Nematoda
Class:	Chromadorea
Order:	Ascaridida
Family:	Toxocaridae
Genus:	Toxocara

Species
Species include:
• Toxocara canis
• Toxocara cati
• Toxocara malaysiensis
• Toxocara tanuki
• Toxocara vitulorum

Transmission

Transmission of *Toxocara* to humans is usually through ingestion of infective eggs. These eggs are passed in cat or dog feces, but the defecation habits of dogs cause *T. canis* transmission to be more common than that of *T. cati*. Both *Toxocara canis* and *Toxocara cati* eggs require a several week incubation period in moist, humid, weather, outside a host before becoming infective, so fresh eggs cannot cause toxocariasis.

Many objects and surfaces can become contaminated with infectious *Toxocara* eggs. Flies that feed on feces can spread *Toxocara* eggs to surfaces or foods. Young children who put contaminated objects in their mouths or eat dirt (pica) are at risk of developing symptoms. Humans can also contaminate foods by not washing their hands before eating.

Humans are not the only accidental hosts of *Toxocara*. Eating undercooked rabbit, chicken, or sheep can lead to infection; encysted larvae in the meat can become reactivated and migrate through a human host, causing toxocariasis. Special attention should be paid to thoroughly cooking giblets and liver to avoid transmission.

Reservoir

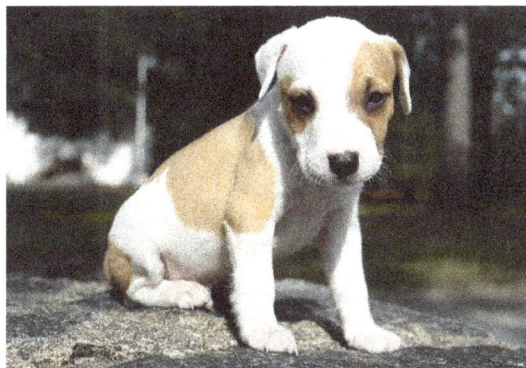

Puppies are the major source of environmental
contamination with roundworm eggs

Dogs and foxes are the reservoir for *Toxocara canis*, but puppies and cubs pose the greatest risk of spreading the infection to humans. Infection in most adult dogs is characterized by encysted second stage larvae. However, these larvae can become reactivated in pregnant females and cross the placental barrier to infect the pups. Vertical transmission can also occur through breastmilk.

Infectious mothers, and puppies under five weeks old, pass eggs in their feces. Approximately 50% of puppies and 20% of adult dogs are infected with *T. canis*.

Cats are the reservoir for *Toxocara cati*. As with *T. canis*, encysted second stage larvae in pregnant or lactating cats become reactivated. However, vertical transmission can only occur through breastfeeding.

Flies can act as mechanical vectors for Toxocara, but most infections occur without a vector. Most incidents with Toxocariasis result from prokaryotic expression vectors and their transmission through direct physical contact with feces that results in the contraction of the illness.

Morphology

Both species produce eggs that are brown and pitted. *T. canis* eggs measure 75-90 μm and are spherical in shape, whereas the eggs of *T. cati* are 65-70 μm in diameter and oblong. Second stage larvae hatch from these eggs and are approximately 0.5mm long and 0.02mm wide. Adults of both species have complete digestive systems and three lips, each composed of a dentigerous ridge.

Adult *T. canis* are found only within dogs and foxes and the males are 4–6 cm in length, with a curved posterior end. The males each have spicules and one "tubular testis." Females can be as long as 15 cm, with the vulva stretching one third of their bodylength. The females do not curve at the posterior end.

T. cati adult females are approximately 10 cm long, while males are typically 6 cm or less. The *T. cati* adults only occur within cats, and male *T. cati* are curved at the posterior end.

Life Cycle

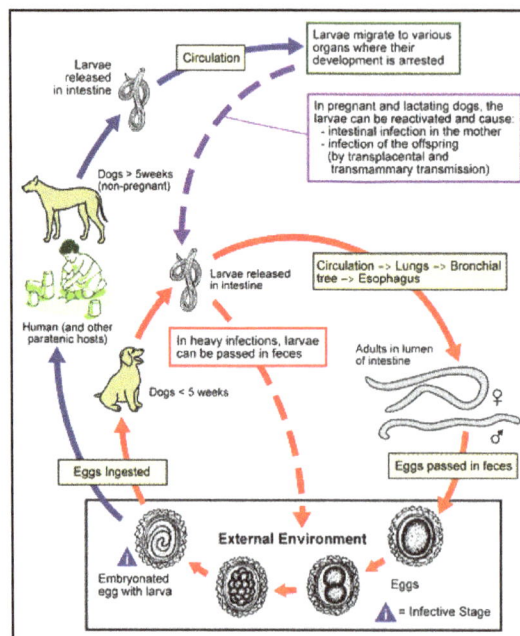

Cats, dogs and foxes can become infected with *Toxocara* through the ingestion of eggs or by transmission of the larvae from a mother to her offspring. Transmission to cats and dogs can also occur by ingestion of infected accidental hosts, such as earthworms, cockroaches, rodents, rabbits, chickens, or sheep.

Eggs hatch as second stage larvae in the intestines of the cat, dog or fox host. Larvae enter the bloodstream and migrate to the lungs, where they are coughed up and swallowed. The larvae mature into adults within the small intestine of a cat, dog or fox, where mating and egg laying occurs. Eggs are passed in the feces and only become infective after several weeks outside of a host. During this incubation period, molting from first to second (and possibly third) stage larva takes place within the egg. In most adult dogs, cats and foxes, the full lifecycle does not occur, but instead second stage larvae encyst after a period of migration through the body. Reactivation of the larvae is common only in pregnant or lactating cats, dogs and foxes. The full lifecycle usually only occurs in these females and their offspring.

Second stage larvae will also hatch in the small intestine of an accidental host, such as a human, after ingestion of infective eggs. The larvae will then migrate through the organs and tissues of the accidental host, most commonly the lungs, liver, eyes, and brain. Since L2 larvae cannot mature in accidental hosts, after this period of migration, *Toxocara* larvae will encyst as second stage larvae.

Diagnosis

Finding *Toxocara* larvae within a patient is the only definitive diagnosis for toxocariasis; however, biopsies to look for second stage larvae in humans are generally not very effective. PCR, ELISA, and serological testing are more commonly used to diagnose *Toxocara* infection. Serological tests are dependent on the number of larvae within the patient, and are unfortunately not very specific. ELISAs are much more reliable and currently have a 78% sensitivity and a 90% specificity. A 2007 study announced an ELISA specific to *Toxocara canis*, which will minimize false positives from cross reactions with similar roundworms and will help distinguish if a patient is infected with *T. canis* or *T. cati*. OLM is often diagnosed after a clinical examination. Granulomas can be found throughout the body and can be visualized using ultrasound, MRI, and CT technologies.

Preventions

Actively involving veterinarians and pet owners is important for controlling the transmission of *Toxocara* from pets to humans. A group very actively involved in promoting a reduction of infections in dogs in the United States is the Companion Animal Parasite Council -- CAPC. Since pregnant or lactating dogs and cats and their offspring have the highest, active parasitic load, these animals should be placed on a deworming program. Pet feces should be picked up and disposed of or buried, as they may contain *Toxocara* eggs. Practicing this measure in public areas, such as parks and beaches, is especially essential for decreasing transmission. Up to 20% of soil samples of U.S. playgrounds have found roundworm eggs. Also, sandboxes should be covered when not in use to prevent cats from using them as litter boxes. Hand washing before eating and after playing with pets, as well as after handling dirt will reduce the chances of ingesting *Toxocara* eggs. Washing all fruits and vegetables, keeping pets out of gardens and thoroughly cooking meats can also prevent transmission. Finally, teaching children not to place nonfood items, especially dirt, in their mouths will drastically reduce the chances of infection.

Toxocariasis has been named one of the neglected diseases of U.S. poverty, because of its prevalence in Appalachia, the southern U.S., inner city settings, and minority populations. Unfortunately, there is currently no vaccine available or under development. However, the mitochondrial genomes of both *T. cati* and *T. canis* have recently been sequenced, which could lead to breakthroughs in treatment and prevention.

Treatment

Toxocariasis will often resolve itself, because the *Toxocara* larvae cannot mature within human hosts. Corticosteroids are prescribed in severe cases of VLM or if the patient is diagnosed with OLM. Either albendazole (preferred) or mebendazole ("second line therapy") may be prescribed. Granulomas can be surgically removed, or laser photocoagulation and cryoretinopexy can be used to destroy ocular granulomas.

Visceral toxocariasis in humans can be treated with antiparasitic drugs such as albendazole or mebendazole, tiabendazole or diethylcarbamazine usually in combination with anti-inflammatory medications. Steroids have been utilized with some positive results. Anti-helminthic therapy is reserved for severe infections (lungs, brain) because therapy may induce, due to massive larval killing, a strong inflammatory response. Treatment of ocular toxocariasis is more difficult and usually consists of measures to prevent progressive damage to the eye.

Other Animals

Cats

Some treatments for infection with *Toxocara cati* include drugs designed to cause the adult worms to become partially anaesthetized and detach from the intestinal lining, allowing them to be excreted live in the feces. Such medications include piperazine and pyrantel. These are frequently combined with the drug praziquantel which appears to cause the worm to lose its resistance to being digested by the host animal. Other effective treatments include ivermectin, milbemycin, and selamectin. Dichlorvos has also been proven to be effective as a poison, though moves to ban it over concerns about its toxicity have made it unavailable in some areas.

Treatment for wild felids, however, is difficult for this parasite, as detection is the best way to find which individuals have the parasite. This can be difficult as infected species are hard to detect. Once detected, the infected individuals would have to be removed from the population, in order to lower the risk of continual exposure to the parasites.

A primary method that has been used to lower the amount of infection is removal through hunting. Removal can also occur through landowners, as Dare and Watkins discovered through their research on cougars. Both hunters and landowners can provide samples that can be used to detect the presence of feline roundworm in the area, as well as help remove it from the population. This method is more practical than administering medications to wild populations, as wild animals, as mentioned before, are harder to find in order to administer medicinal care.

Medicinal care, however, is also another method used in round worm studies; such as the experiment on managing raccoon roundworm done by Smyser et al. in which they implemented medical baiting. However, medicine is often expensive and the success of the baiting depends on if the infected individuals consume the bait. Additionally, it can be costly (in time and resources) to check on baited areas. Removal by hunting allows agencies to reduce costs and gives agencies a more improved chance of removing infected individuals.

Rocky Mountain Spotted Fever

Rocky Mountain spotted fever (RMSF) is a bacterial disease spread by ticks. It typically begins with a fever and headache, which is followed a few days later with the development of a rash. The rash is generally made up of small spots of bleeding and starts on the wrists and ankles. Other symptoms may include muscle pains and vomiting. Long-term complications following recovery may include hearing loss or loss of part of an arm or leg.

The disease is caused by *Rickettsia rickettsii*, a type of bacterium that is primarily spread to humans by American dog ticks, Rocky Mountain wood ticks, and brown dog ticks. Rarely the disease is spread by blood transfusions. Diagnosis in the early stages is difficult. A number of laboratory tests can confirm the diagnosis but treatment should be begun based on symptoms. It is within a group known as spotted fever rickettsiosis, together with *Rickettsia parkeri* rickettsiosis, Pacific Coast tick fever, and rickettsialpox.

Treatment of RMSF is with the antibiotic doxycycline. It works best when started early and is recommended in all age groups, as well as during pregnancy. Antibiotics are not recommended for prevention. Approximately 0.5% of people who are infected die as a result. Before the discovery of tetracycline in the 1940s, more than 10% of those with RMSF died.

Less than 5,000 cases are reported a year in the United States, most often in June and July. It has been diagnosed throughout the contiguous United States, Western Canada, and parts of Central and South America. Rocky Mountain spotted fever was first identified in the 1800s in the Rocky Mountains.

Signs and Symptoms

Spotted fever can be very difficult to diagnose in its early stages, due to the similarity of symptoms with many different diseases.

People infected with *R. rickettsii* usually notice symptoms following an incubation period of one to two weeks after a tick bite. The early clinical presentation of Rocky Mountain spotted fever is nonspecific and may resemble a variety of other infectious and noninfectious diseases.

Initial symptoms:

- Fever
- Nausea
- Emesis (vomiting)
- Severe headache

- Muscle pain

- Lack of appetite

- Parotitis in some cases (somewhat rare).

Later signs and symptoms:

- Maculopapular rash

- Petechial rash

- Abdominal pain

- Joint pain

- Conjunctivitis

- Forgetfulness.

The classic triad of findings for this disease are fever, rash, and history of tick bite. However, this combination is often not identified when the people initially presents for care. The rash has a centripetal, or "inward" pattern of spread, meaning it begins at the extremities and courses towards the trunk.

Rash

The rash first appears two to five days after the onset of fever, and it is often quite subtle. Younger patients usually develop the rash earlier than older patients. Most often the rash begins as small, flat, pink, nonitchy spots (macules) on the wrists, forearms, and ankles. These spots turn pale when pressure is applied and eventually become raised on the skin. The characteristic red, spotted (petechial) rash of Rocky Mountain spotted fever is usually not seen until the sixth day or later after onset of symptoms, but this type of rash occurs in only 35 to 60% of patients with Rocky Mountain spotted fever. The rash involves the palms or soles in as many as 80% of people. However, this distribution may not occur until later on in the course of the disease. As many as 15% of patients may never develop a rash.

Complications

People can develop permanent disabilities including "cognitive deficits, ataxia, hemiparesis, blindness, deafness, or amputation following gangrene".

Cause

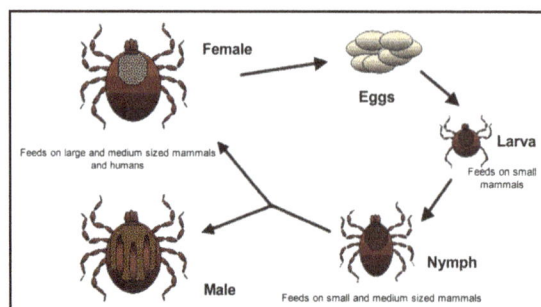

The lifecycle of *Dermacentor variabilis* and *Dermacentor andersoni* ticks (Family Ixodidae)

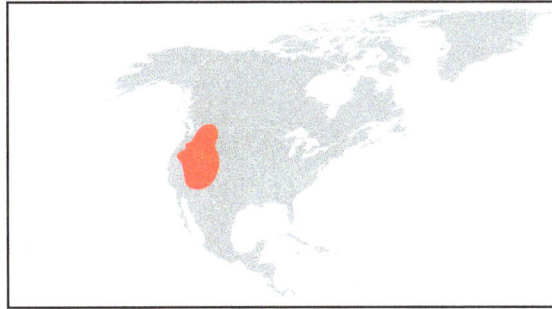
American dog tick (*Dermacentor variabilis*) range

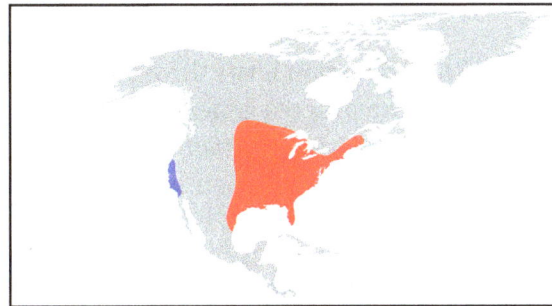
Rocky Mountain wood tick (Dermacentor andersoni) range

Ticks are the natural hosts of the disease, serving as both reservoirs and vectors of *R. rickettsii* Ticks transmit the bacteria primarily by their bites. Less commonly, infections may occur following exposure to crushed tick tissues, fluids, or tick feces.

A female tick can transmit *R. rickettsii* to her eggs in a process called transovarial transmission. Ticks can also become infected with *R. rickettsii* while feeding on blood from the host in either the larval or nymphal stage. After the tick develops into the next stage, the *R. rickettsii* may be transmitted to the second host during the feeding process. Furthermore, male ticks may transfer *R. rickettsii* to female ticks through body fluids or spermatozoa during the mating process. These types of transmission represent how generations or life stages of infected ticks are maintained. Once infected, the tick can carry the pathogen for life.

Rickettsiae are transmitted to through saliva injected while a tick is feeding. Unlike Lyme disease and other tick-borne pathogens that require a prolonged attachment period to establish infection, a person can become infected with *R. rickettsii* in a feeding time as short as 2 hours. In general, about 1-3% of the tick population carries *R. rickettsii*, even in areas where the majority of human cases are reported. Therefore, the risk of exposure to a tick carrying *R. rickettsii* is low.

The disease is spread by the American dog tick (*Dermacentor variabilis*), Rocky Mountain wood tick (*D. andersoni)*, brown dog tick (*Rhipicephalus sanguineus*), and *Amblyomma sculptum*. Not all of these are of equal importance, and most are restricted to certain geographic areas.

The two major vectors of *R. rickettsii* in the United States are the American dog tick and the Rocky Mountain wood tick. American dog ticks are widely distributed east of the Rocky Mountains and they also occur in limited areas along the Pacific Coast. Dogs and medium-sized mammals are the preferred hosts of an adult American dog tick, although it feeds readily on other large mammals, including human beings. This tick is the most commonly identified species responsible for transmitting *R. rickettsii* to humans. Rocky Mountain wood ticks (*D. andersoni*) are found in the Rocky

Mountain states and in southwestern Canada. The lifecycle of this tick may require up to three years for its completion. The adult ticks feed primarily on large mammals. The larvae and nymphs feed on small rodents.

Other tick species have been shown to be naturally infected with *R. rickettsii* or serve as experimental vectors in the laboratory. These species are likely to play only a minor role in the ecology of *R. rickettsii*.

Pathophysiology

Entry into Host

Rickettsia rickettsii can be transmitted to human hosts through the bite of an infected tick. As with other bacterium transmitted via ticks, the process generally requires a period of attachment of 4 to 6 hours. However, in some cases a *Rickettsia rickettsii* infection has been contracted by contact with tick tissues or fluids. Then, the bacteria induce their internalization into host cells via a receptor-mediated invasion mechanism.

Researchers believe that this mechanism is similar to that of *Rickettsia conorii*. This species of *Rickettsia* uses an abundant cell surface protein called OmpB to attach to a host cell membrane protein called Ku70. It has previously been reported that Ku70 migrates to the host cell surface in the presence of "Rickettsia". Then, Ku70 is ubiquitinated by c-Cbl, an E3 ubiquitin ligase. This triggers a cascade of signal transduction events resulting in the recruitment of Arp2/3 complex. CDC42, protein tyrosine kinase, phosphoinositide 3-kinase, and Src-family kinases then activate Arp2/3. This causes the alteration of local host cytoskeletal actin at the entry site as part of a zipper mechanism. Then, the bacteria is phagocytosized by the host cell and enveloped by a phagosome.

Studies have suggested that rOmpB is involved in this process of adhesion and invasion. Both rOmpA and rOmpB are members of a family of surface cell antigens (Sca) which are autotransporter proteins; they act as ligands for the Omp proteins and are found throughout the *rickettsiae*.

Exit from Host Cell

The cytosol of the host cell contains nutrients, adenosine triphosphate, amino acids, and nucleotides which are used by the bacteria for growth. For this reason, as well as to avoid phagolysosomal fusion and death, rickettsiae must escape from the phagosome. To escape from the phagosome, the bacteria secrete phospholipase D and hemolysin C. This causes disruption of the phagosomal membrane and allows the bacteria to escape. Following generation time in the cytoplasm of the host cells, the bacteria utilizes actin based motility to move through the cytosol.

RickA, expressed on the rickettsial surface, activates Arp2/3 and causes actin polymerization. The rickettsiae use the actin to propel themselves throughout the cytosol to the surface of the host cell. This causes the host cell membrane to protrude outward and invaginate the membrane of an adjacent cell. The bacteria are then taken up by the neighboring cell in a double membrane vacuole that the bacteria can subsequently lyse, enabling spread from cell to cell without exposure to the extracellular environment.

Consequences of Infection

Rickettsia rickettsii initially infect blood vessel endothelial cells, but eventually migrate to vital organs such as the brain, skin, and the heart via the blood stream. Bacterial replication in host cells causes endothelial cell proliferation and inflammation, resulting in mononuclear cell infiltration into blood vessels and subsequent red blood cell leakage into surrounding tissues. The characteristic rash observed in Rocky Mountain spotted fever is the direct result of this localized replication of rickettsia in blood vessel endothelial cells.

Diagnosis

Even doctors who are familiar with the disease find it hard to diagnose early during infection.

Abnormal laboratory findings seen in patients with Rocky Mountain spotted fever may include a low platelet count, low blood sodium concentration, or elevated liver enzyme levels. Serology testing and skin biopsy are considered to be the best methods of diagnosis. Although immuno-fluorescent antibody assays are considered some of the best serology tests available, most antibodies that fight against *R. rickettsii* are undetectable on serology tests the first seven days after infection.

Differential diagnosis includes dengue, leptospirosis, chikungunya, and Zika fever.

Treatment

Appropriate antibiotic treatment should be started immediately when there is a suspicion of Rocky Mountain spotted fever. Early treatment of Rocky Mountain spotted fever prevents further damage to internal organs. Treatment should not be delayed for laboratory confirmation. Failure to respond to a tetracycline argues against a diagnosis of Rocky Mountain spotted fever. Severely ill people may require longer periods before their fever resolves, especially if they have experienced damage to multiple organ systems. Preventive therapy in healthy people who have had recent tick bites is not recommended and may only delay the onset of disease.

Doxycycline (a tetracycline) is the drug of choice for patients with Rocky Mountain spotted fever, being one of the only instances doxycycline is used in children. Treatment typically consists of 100 milligrams every 12 hours, or for children under 45 kg (99 lb) at 4 mg/kg of body weight per day in two divided doses. Treatment should be continued for at least three days after the fever subsides, and until there is unequivocal evidence of clinical improvement. This will be generally for a minimum time of five to ten days. Severe or complicated outbreaks may require longer treatment courses. Doxycycline/ tetracycline is also the preferred drug for patients with ehrlichiosis, another tick-transmitted infection with signs and symptoms that may resemble those of Rocky Mountain spotted fever. Chloramphenicol is an alternative drug that can be used to treat Rocky Mountain spotted fever, specifically in pregnancy. However, this drug may be associated with a wide range of side effects, and careful monitoring of blood levels is required.

Prognosis

Rocky Mountain spotted fever can be a very severe illness and patients often require hospitalization. Because *R. rickettsii* infects the cells lining blood vessels throughout the body, severe manifestations of this disease may involve the respiratory system, central nervous system, gastro-intestinal system, or kidneys.

Long-term health problems following acute Rocky Mountain spotted fever infection include partial paralysis of the lower extremities, gangrene requiring amputation of fingers, toes, or arms or legs, hearing loss, loss of bowel or bladder control, movement disorders, and language disorders. These complications are most frequent in persons recovering from severe, life-threatening disease, often following lengthy hospitalizations.

Swine Influenza

Swine influenza is an infection caused by any one of several types of swine influenza viruses. Swine influenza virus (SIV) or swine-origin influenza virus (S-OIV) is any strain of the influenza family of viruses that is endemic in pigs. As of 2009, the known SIV strains include influenza C and the subtypes of influenza A known as H1N1, H1N2, H2N1, H3N1, H3N2, and H2N3.

The Swine flu was initially seen in humans in Mexico in 2009, where the strain of the particular virus was a mixture from 3 types of strains. Six of the genes are very similar to the H1N2 influenza virus that was found in pigs around 2000.

Swine influenza virus is common throughout pig populations worldwide. Transmission of the virus from pigs to humans is not common and does not always lead to human flu, often resulting only in the production of antibodies in the blood. If transmission does cause human flu, it is called zoonotic swine flu. People with regular exposure to pigs are at increased risk of swine flu infection.

Around the mid-20th century, identification of influenza subtypes became possible, allowing accurate diagnosis of transmission to humans. Since then, only 50 such transmissions have been confirmed. These strains of swine flu rarely pass from human to human. Symptoms of zoonotic swine flu in humans are similar to those of influenza and of influenza-like illness in general, namely chills, fever, sore throat, muscle pains, severe headache, coughing, weakness, shortness of breath, and general discomfort.

In August 2010, the World Health Organization declared the swine flu pandemic officially over.

Signs and Symptoms

In swine flu, an influenza infection produces fever, lethargy, sneezing, coughing, difficulty breathing and decreased appetite. In some cases the infection can cause miscarriage. Although mortality is usually low (around 1–4%), the virus can produce weight loss and poor growth, causing economic loss to farmers. Infected pigs can lose up to 12 pounds of body weight over a three- to four-week period. Swine have receptors to which both avian and mammalian influenza viruses are able to bind to, which leads to the virus being able to evolve and mutate into different forms. Influenza A is responsible for infecting swine, and was first identified in the summer of 1918. Pigs have often been seen as "mixing vessels", which help to change and evolve strains of disease that are then passed on to other mammals, such as humans.

Humans

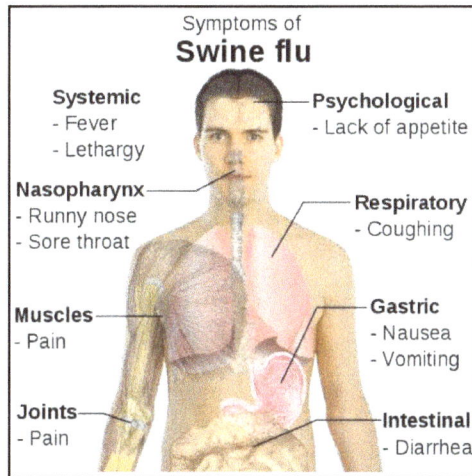

Main symptoms of swine flu in humans

Direct transmission of a swine flu virus from pigs to humans is occasionally possible (zoonotic swine flu). In all, 50 cases are known to have occurred since the first report in medical literature in 1958, which have resulted in a total of six deaths. Of these six people, one was pregnant, one had leukemia, one had Hodgkin's lymphoma and two were known to be previously healthy. One of these had unknown whereabouts. Despite these apparently low numbers of infections, the true rate of infection may be higher, since most cases only cause a very mild disease, and will probably never be reported or diagnosed.

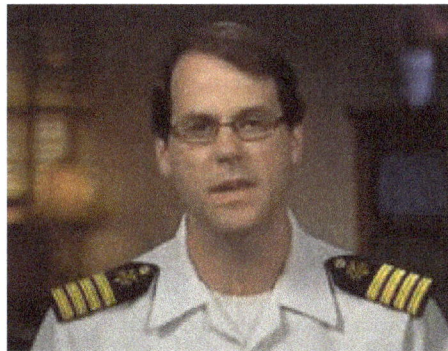

Dr. Joe Bresee, with CDC's Influenza Division, describes the symptoms of swine flu and warning signs to look for that indicate the need for urgent medical attention

According to the Centers for Disease Control and Prevention (CDC), in humans the symptoms of the 2009 "swine flu" H1N1 virus are similar to those of influenza and of influenza-like illness in general. Symptoms include fever; cough, sore throat, watery eyes, body aches, shortness of breath, headache, weight loss, chills, sneezing, runny nose, coughing, dizziness, abdominal pain, lack of appetite and fatigue. The 2009 outbreak has shown an increased percentage of patients reporting diarrhea and vomiting as well. The 2009 H1N1 virus is not zoonotic swine flu, as it is not transmitted from pigs to humans, but from person to person through airborne droplets.

Because these symptoms are not specific to swine flu, a differential diagnosis of *probable* swine flu requires not only symptoms, but also a high likelihood of swine flu due to the person's recent and past medical history. For example, during the 2009 swine flu outbreak in the United States, the CDC advised physicians to "consider swine influenza infection in the differential diagnosis of patients with acute febrile respiratory illness who have either been in contact with persons with confirmed swine flu, or who were in one of the five U.S. states that have reported swine flu cases or in Mexico during the seven days preceding their illness onset." A diagnosis of *confirmed* swine flu requires laboratory testing of a respiratory sample (a simple nose and throat swab).

The most common cause of death is respiratory failure. Other causes of death are pneumonia (leading to sepsis), high fever (leading to neurological problems), dehydration (from excessive vomiting and diarrhea), electrolyte imbalance and kidney failure. Fatalities are more likely in young children and the elderly.

Virology

Transmission between Pigs

Influenza is quite common in pigs, with about half of breeding pigs having been exposed to the virus in the US. Antibodies to the virus are also common in pigs in other countries.

The main route of transmission is through direct contact between infected and uninfected animals. These close contacts are particularly common during animal transport. Intensive farming may also increase the risk of transmission, as the pigs are raised in very close proximity to each other. The direct transfer of the virus probably occurs either by pigs touching noses, or through dried mucus. Airborne transmission through the aerosols produced by pigs coughing or sneezing are also an important means of infection. The virus usually spreads quickly through a herd, infecting all the pigs within just a few days. Transmission may also occur through wild animals, such as wild boar, which can spread the disease between farms.

To Humans

People who work with poultry and swine, especially those with intense exposures, are at increased risk of zoonotic infection with influenza virus endemic in these animals, and constitute a population of human hosts in which zoonosis and reassortment can co-occur. Vaccination of these workers against influenza and surveillance for new influenza strains among this population may therefore be an important public health measure. Transmission of influenza from swine to humans who work with swine was documented in a small surveillance study performed in 2004 at the University of Iowa. This study, among others, forms the basis of a recommendation that people whose jobs involve handling poultry and swine be the focus of increased public health surveillance. Other professions at particular risk of infection are veterinarians and meat processing workers, although the risk of infection for both of these groups is lower than that of farm workers.

Interaction with Avian H5N1 in Pigs

Pigs are unusual as they can be infected with influenza strains that usually infect three different species: pigs, birds and humans. This makes pigs a host where influenza viruses might exchange genes, producing new and dangerous strains. Avian influenza virus H3N2 is endemic in pigs in China, and has been detected in pigs in Vietnam, increasing fears of the emergence of new variant strains. H3N2 evolved from H2N2 by antigenic shift. In August 2004, researchers in China found

H5N1 in pigs.

These H5N1 infections may be quite common; in a survey of 10 apparently healthy pigs housed near poultry farms in West Java, where avian flu had broken out, five of the pig samples contained the H5N1 virus. The Indonesian government has since found similar results in the same region. Additional tests of 150 pigs outside the area were negative.

Structure

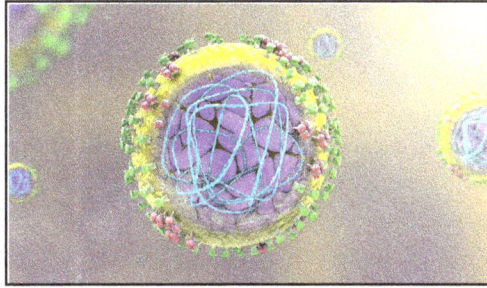

Structure of H1N1 Virion

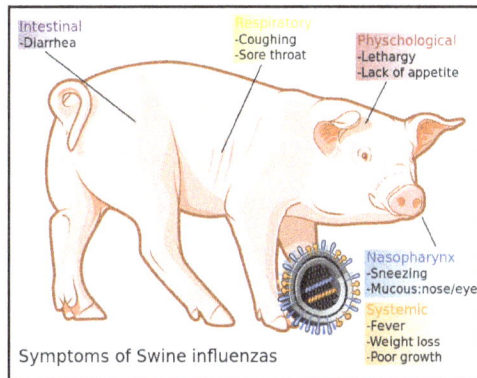

Main symptoms of swine flu in swine

The influenza virion is roughly spherical. It is an enveloped virus; the outer layer is a lipid membrane which is taken from the host cell in which the virus multiplies. Inserted into the lipid membrane are "spikes", which are proteins—actually glycoproteins, because they consist of protein linked to sugars—known as HA (hemagglutinin) and NA (neuraminidase). These are the proteins that determine the subtype of influenza virus (A/H1N1, for example). The HA and NA are important in the immune response against the virus; antibodies (proteins made to combat infection) against these spikes may protect against infection. The NA protein is the target of the antiviral drugs Relenza and Tamiflu. Also embedded in the lipid membrane is the M2 protein, which is the target of the antiviral adamantanes amantadine and rimantadine.

Classification

Of the three genera of influenza viruses that cause human flu, two also cause influenza in pigs, with influenza A being common in pigs and influenza C being rare. Influenza B has not been reported in pigs. Within influenza A and influenza C, the strains found in pigs and humans are largely distinct, although because of reassortment there have been transfers of genes among strains crossing swine, avian, and human species boundaries.

Influenza C

Influenza viruses infect both humans and pigs, but do not infect birds. Transmission between pigs and humans have occurred in the past. For example, influenza C caused small outbreaks of a mild form of influenza amongst children in Japan and California. Because of its limited host range and the lack of genetic diversity in influenza C, this form of influenza does not cause pandemics in humans.

Influenza A

Swine influenza is caused by influenza A subtypes H1N1, H1N2, H2N3, H3N1, and H3N2. In pigs, four influenza A virus subtypes (H1N1, H1N2, H3N2 and H7N9) are the most common strains worldwide. In the United States, the H1N1 subtype was exclusively prevalent among swine populations before 1998; however, since late August 1998, H3N2 subtypes have been isolated from pigs. As of 2004, H3N2 virus isolates in US swine and turkey stocks were triple reassortants, containing genes from human (HA, NA, and PB1), swine (NS, NP, and M), and avian (PB2 and PA) lineages. In August 2012, the Center for Disease Control and Prevention confirmed 145 human cases (113 in Indiana, 30 in Ohio, one in Hawaii and one in Illinois) of H3N2v since July 2012. The death of a 61-year-old Madison County, Ohio woman is the first in the nation associated with a new swine flu strain. She contracted the illness after having contact with hogs at the Ross County Fair.

Diagnosis

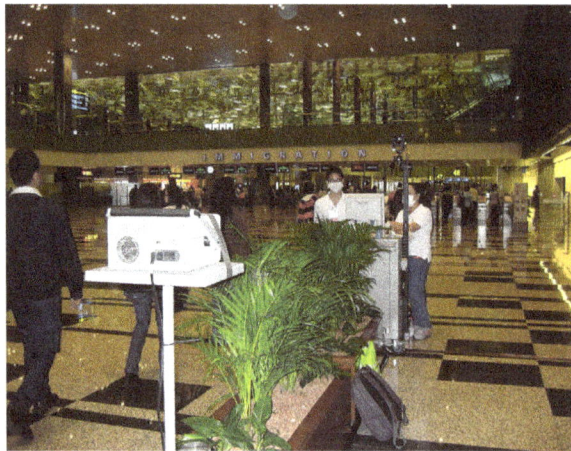

Thermal scanning of passengers arriving at Singapore Changi airport

The CDC recommends real-time PCR as the method of choice for diagnosing H1N1. The oral or nasal fluid collection and RNA virus preserving filter paper card is commercially available. This method allows a specific diagnosis of novel influenza (H1N1) as opposed to seasonal influenza. Near-patient point-of-care tests are in development.

Prevention

Prevention of swine influenza has three components: prevention in pigs, prevention of transmission to humans, and prevention of its spread among humans. Proper hand washing techniques can prevent the virus from spreading. By washing hands often, for about as long as one can sing the happy birthday song twice. Avoid touching the eyes, nose or mouth. Stay away from others who display symptoms of the cold or flu, and also avoid contact with others when displaying symptoms.

Swine

Methods of preventing the spread of influenza among swine include facility management, herd management, and vaccination (ATCvet code: QI09AA03 (WHO)). Because much of the illness and death associated with swine flu involves secondary infection by other pathogens, control strategies that rely on vaccination may be insufficient.

Control of swine influenza by vaccination has become more difficult in recent decades, as the evolution of the virus has resulted in inconsistent responses to traditional vaccines. Standard commercial swine flu vaccines are effective in controlling the infection when the virus strains match enough to have significant cross-protection, and custom (autogenous) vaccines made from the specific viruses isolated are created and used in the more difficult cases. Present vaccination strategies for SIV control and prevention in swine farms typically include the use of one of several bivalent SIV vaccines commercially available in the United States. Of the 97 recent H3N2 isolates examined, only 41 isolates had strong serologic cross-reactions with antiserum to three commercial SIV vaccines. Since the protective ability of influenza vaccines depends primarily on the closeness of the match between the vaccine virus and the epidemic virus, the presence of nonreactive H3N2 SIV variants suggests current commercial vaccines might not effectively protect pigs from infection with a majority of H3N2 viruses. The United States Department of Agriculture researchers say while pig vaccination keeps pigs from getting sick, it does not block infection or shedding of the virus.

Facility management includes using disinfectants and ambient temperature to control viruses in the environment. They are unlikely to survive outside living cells for more than two weeks, except in cold (but above freezing) conditions, and are readily inactivated by disinfectants. Herd management includes not adding pigs carrying influenza to herds that have not been exposed to the virus. The virus survives in healthy carrier pigs for up to three months, and can be recovered from them between outbreaks. Carrier pigs are usually responsible for the introduction of SIV into previously uninfected herds and countries, so new animals should be quarantined. After an outbreak, as immunity in exposed pigs wanes, new outbreaks of the same strain can occur.

Humans

Prevention of pig-to-human Transmission

The transmission from swine to humans is believed to occur mainly in swine farms, where farmers are in close contact with live pigs. Although strains of swine influenza are usually not able to infect humans, this may occasionally happen, so farmers and veterinarians are encouraged to use face masks when dealing with infected animals. The use of vaccines on swine to prevent their infection is a major method of limiting swine-to-human transmission. Risk factors that may contribute to swine-to-human transmission include smoking and, especially, not wearing gloves when working with sick animals, thereby increasing the likelihood of subsequent hand-to-eye, hand-to-nose or hand-to-mouth transmission.

Swine can be infected by both avian and human flu strains of influenza, and therefore are
hosts where the antigenic shifts can occur that create new influenza strains

Prevention of Human-to-human Transmission

Influenza spreads between humans when infected people cough or sneeze, then other people
breathe in the virus or touch something with the virus on it and then touch their own face. "Avoid
touching your eyes, nose or mouth. Germs spread this way." Swine flu cannot be spread by pork
products, since the virus is not transmitted through food. The swine flu in humans is most contagious during the first five days of the illness, although some people, most commonly children,
can remain contagious for up to ten days. Diagnosis can be made by sending a specimen, collected
during the first five days, for analysis.

Thermal imaging camera and screen, photographed in an airport terminal in Greece – thermal imaging
can detect elevated body temperature, one of the signs of the virus H1N1 (swine influenza)

Recommendations to prevent spread of the virus among humans include using standard infection
control, which includes frequent washing of hands with soap and water or with alcohol-based hand

sanitizers, especially after being out in public. Chance of transmission is also reduced by disinfecting household surfaces, which can be done effectively with a diluted chlorine bleach solution.

Experts agree hand-washing can help prevent viral infections, including ordinary and the swine flu infections. Also, avoiding touching one's eyes, nose or mouth with one's hands helps to prevent the flu. Influenza can spread in coughs or sneezes, but an increasing body of evidence shows small droplets containing the virus can linger on tabletops, telephones and other surfaces and be transferred via the fingers to the eyes, nose or mouth. Alcohol-based gel or foam hand sanitizers work well to destroy viruses and bacteria. Anyone with flu-like symptoms, such as a sudden fever, cough or muscle aches, should stay away from work or public transportation, and should contact a doctor for advice.

Social distancing, another tactic, is staying away from other people who might be infected, and can include avoiding large gatherings, spreading out a little at work, or perhaps staying home and lying low if an infection is spreading in a community. Public health and other responsible authorities have action plans which may request or require social distancing actions, depending on the severity of the outbreak.

Vaccination

Vaccines are available for different kinds of swine flu. The U.S. Food and Drug Administration (FDA) approved the new swine flu vaccine for use in the United States on September 15, 2009. Studies by the National Institutes of Health show a single dose creates enough antibodies to protect against the virus within about 10 days.

In the aftermath of the 2009 pandemic, several studies were conducted to see who received influenza vaccines. These studies show that whites are much more likely to be vaccinated for seasonal influenza and for the H1N1 strain than African Americans This could be due to several factors. Historically, there has been mistrust of vaccines and of the medical community from African Americans. Many African Americans do not believe vaccines or doctors to be effective. This mistrust stems from the exploitation of the African American communities during studies like the Tuskegee study. Additionally, vaccines are typically administered in clinics, hospitals, or doctor's offices. Many people of lower socioeconomic status are less likely to receive vaccinations because they do not have health insurance.

Surveillance

Although there is no formal national surveillance system in the United States to determine what viruses are circulating in pigs, an informal surveillance network in the United States is part of a world surveillance network.

Treatment

Swine

As swine influenza is rarely fatal to pigs, little treatment beyond rest and supportive care is required. Instead, veterinary efforts are focused on preventing the spread of the virus throughout the farm, or to other farms. Vaccination and animal management techniques are most important in these efforts. Antibiotics are also used to treat this disease, which although they have no effect against the influenza virus, do help prevent bacterial pneumonia and other secondary infections in influenza-weakened herds.

In Europe the avian-like H1N1 and the human-like H3N2 and H1N2 are the most common influenza subtypes in swine, of which avian-like H1N1 is the most frequent. Since 2009 another subtype, pdmH1N1, emerged globally and also in European pig population. The prevalence varies from country to country but all of the subtypes are continuously circulating in swine herds. In the EU region whole-virus vaccines are available which are inactivated and adjuvanted. Vaccination of sows is common practice and reveals also a benefit to young pigs by prolonging the maternally level of antibodies. Several commercial vaccines are available including a trivalent one being used in sow vaccination and a vaccine against pdmH1N1. In vaccinated sows multiplication of viruses and virus shedding are significantly reduced.

Humans

If a person becomes sick with swine flu, antiviral drugs can make the illness milder and make the patient feel better faster. They may also prevent serious flu complications. For treatment, antiviral drugs work best if started soon after getting sick (within two days of symptoms). Beside antivirals, supportive care at home or in a hospital focuses on controlling fevers, relieving pain and maintaining fluid balance, as well as identifying and treating any secondary infections or other medical problems. The U.S. Centers for Disease Control and Prevention recommends the use of oseltamivir (Tamiflu) or zanamivir (Relenza) for the treatment and/or prevention of infection with swine influenza viruses; however, the majority of people infected with the virus make a full recovery without requiring medical attention or antiviral drugs. The virus isolated in the 2009 outbreak have been found resistant to amantadine and rimantadine.

In the U.S., on April 27, 2009, the FDA issued Emergency use Authorizations to make available Relenza and Tamiflu antiviral drugs to treat the swine influenza virus in cases for which they are currently unapproved. The agency issued these EUAs to allow treatment of patients younger than the current approval allows and to allow the widespread distribution of the drugs, including by volunteers.

Lyme Disease

Lyme disease, also known as Lyme borreliosis, is an infectious disease caused by the *Borrelia* bacterium which is spread by ticks. The most common sign of infection is an expanding area of redness on the skin, known as erythema migrans, that appears at the site of the tick bite about a week after it occurred. The rash is typically neither itchy nor painful. Approximately 70–80% of infected people develop a rash. Other early symptoms may include fever, headache and tiredness. If untreated, symptoms may include loss of the ability to move one or both sides of the face, joint pains, severe headaches with neck stiffness, or heart palpitations, among others. Months to years later, repeated episodes of joint pain and swelling may occur. Occasionally, people develop shooting pains or tingling in their arms and legs. Despite appropriate treatment, about 10 to 20%

of people develop joint pains, memory problems, and tiredness for at least six months.

Lyme disease is transmitted to humans by the bites of infected ticks of the genus *Ixodes*. In the United States, ticks of concern are usually of the *Ixodes scapularis* type, and must be attached for at least 36 hours before the bacteria can spread. In Europe ticks of the *Ixodes ricinus* type may spread the bacteria more quickly. In North America, *Borrelia burgdorferi* and *Borrelia mayonii* are the cause. In Europe and Asia, the bacteria *Borrelia afzelii* and *Borrelia garinii* are also causes of the disease. The disease does not appear to be transmissible between people, by other animals, or through food. Diagnosis is based upon a combination of symptoms, history of tick exposure, and possibly testing for specific antibodies in the blood. Blood tests are often negative in the early stages of the disease. Testing of individual ticks is not typically useful.

Prevention includes efforts to prevent tick bites such as by wearing clothing to cover the arms and legs, and using DEET-based insect repellents. Using pesticides to reduce tick numbers may also be effective. Ticks can be removed using tweezers. If the removed tick was full of blood, a single dose of doxycycline may be used to prevent development of infection, but is not generally recommended since development of infection is rare. If an infection develops, a number of antibiotics are effective, including doxycycline, amoxicillin, and cefuroxime. Standard treatment usually lasts for two or three weeks. Some people develop a fever and muscle and joint pains from treatment which may last for one or two days. In those who develop persistent symptoms, long-term antibiotic therapy has not been found to be useful.

Lyme disease is the most common disease spread by ticks in the Northern Hemisphere. It is estimated to affect 300,000 people a year in the United States and 65,000 people a year in Europe. Infections are most common in the spring and early summer. Lyme disease was diagnosed as a separate condition for the first time in 1975 in Old Lyme, Connecticut. It was originally mistaken for juvenile rheumatoid arthritis. The bacterium involved was first described in 1981 by Willy Burgdorfer. Chronic symptoms following treatment are well described and are known as "post-treatment Lyme disease syndrome" (PTLDS). PTLDS is different from chronic Lyme disease; a term no longer supported by the scientific community and used in different ways by different groups. Some healthcare providers claim that PTLDS is caused by persistent infection, but this is not believed to be true because of the inability to detect infectious organisms after standard treatment. A vaccine for Lyme disease was marketed in the United States between 1998 and 2002, but was withdrawn from the market due to poor sales. Research is ongoing to develop new vaccines.

Signs and Symptoms

Lyme disease can affect multiple body systems and produce a broad range of symptoms. Not everyone with Lyme disease have all symptoms, and many of the symptoms are not specific to Lyme disease, but can occur with other diseases, as well.

The incubation period from infection to the onset of symptoms is usually one to two weeks, but can be much shorter (days), or much longer (months to years). Lyme symptoms most often occur from May to September, because the nymphal stage of the tick is responsible for most cases. Asymptomatic infection exists, but occurs in less than 7% of infected individuals in the United States. Asymptomatic infection may be much more common among those infected in Europe.

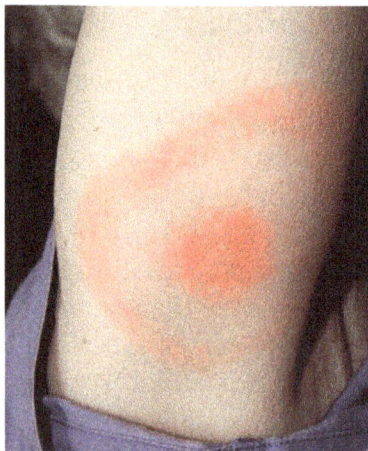

An expanding rash is an initial sign of about 80% of Lyme infections. The rash may look like a "bull's eye," as pictured, in about 80% of cases in Europe and 20% of cases in the US

Early Localized Infection

Early localized infection can occur when the infection has not yet spread throughout the body. Only the site where the infection has first come into contact with the skin is affected. The initial sign of about 80% of Lyme infections is an Erythema migrans (EM) rash at the site of a tick bite, often near skin folds, such as the armpit, groin, or back of knee, on the trunk, under clothing straps, or in children's hair, ear, or neck. Most people who get infected do not remember seeing a tick or the bite. The rash appears typically one or two weeks (range 3–32 days) after the bite and expands 2–3 cm per day up to a diameter of 5–70 cm (median 16 cm). The rash is usually circular or oval, red or bluish, and may have an elevated or darker center. In about 79% of cases in Europe but only 19% of cases in endemic areas of the U.S., the rash gradually clears from the center toward the edges, possibly forming a "bull's eye" pattern. The rash may feel warm but usually is not itchy, is rarely tender or painful, and takes up to four weeks to resolve if untreated.

The EM rash is often accompanied by symptoms of a viral-like illness, including fatigue, headache, body aches, fever, and chills, but usually not nausea or upper-respiratory problems. These symptoms may also appear without a rash, or linger after the rash disappears. Lyme can progress to later stages without these symptoms or a rash.

People with high fever for more than two days or whose other symptoms of viral-like illness do not improve despite antibiotic treatment for Lyme disease, or who have abnormally low levels of white or red cells or platelets in the blood, should be investigated for possible coinfection with other tick-borne diseases, such as ehrlichiosis and babesiosis.

Early Disseminated Infection

Within days to weeks after the onset of local infection, the *Borrelia* bacteria may spread through the lymphatic system or bloodstream. In 10-20% of untreated cases, EM rashes develop at sites across the body that bear no relation to the original tick bite. Transient muscle pains and joint pains are also common.

In about 10-15% of untreated people, Lyme causes neurological problems known as neuroborreliosis.

Early neuroborreliosis typically appears 4–6 weeks (range 1–12 weeks) after the tick bite and involves some combination of lymphocytic meningitis, cranial neuritis, radiculopathy and/or mononeuritis multiplex. Lymphocytic meningitis causes characteristic changes in the cerebrospinal fluid (CSF) and may be accompanied for several weeks by variable headache and, less commonly, usually mild meningitis signs such as inability to flex the neck fully and intolerance to bright lights, but typically no or only very low fever. In children, partial loss of vision may also occur. Cranial neuritis is an inflammation of cranial nerves. When due to Lyme, it most typically causes facial palsy impairing blinking, smiling, and chewing in one or both sides of the face. It may also cause intermittent double vision. Lyme radiculopathy is an inflammation of spinal nerve roots that often causes pain and less often weakness, numbness, or altered sensation in the areas of the body served by nerves connected to the affected roots, e.g. limb(s) or part(s) of trunk. The pain is often described as unlike any other previously felt, excruciating, migrating, worse at night, rarely symmetrical, and often accompanied by extreme sleep disturbance. Mononeuritis multiplex is an inflammation causing similar symptoms in one or more unrelated peripheral nerves. Rarely, early neuroborreliosis may involve inflammation of the brain or spinal cord, with symptoms such as confusion, abnormal gait, ocular movements, or speech, impaired movement, impaired motor planning, or shaking.

In North America, facial palsy is the typical early neuroborreliosis presentation, occurring in 5-10% of untreated people, in about 75% of cases accompanied by lymphocytic meningitis. Lyme radiculopathy is reported half as frequently, but many cases may be unrecognized. In European adults, the most common presentation is a combination of lymphocytic meningitis and radiculopathy known as Bannwarth syndrome, accompanied in 36-89% of cases by facial palsy. In this syndrome, radicular pain tends to start in the same body region as the initial erythema migrans rash, if there was one, and precedes possible facial palsy and other impaired movement. In extreme cases, permanent impairment of motor or sensory function of the lower limbs may occur. In European children, the most common manifestations are facial palsy (in 55%), other cranial neuritis, and lymphocytic meningitis (in 27%).

In about 4-10% of untreated cases in the U.S. and 0.3-4% of untreated cases in Europe, typically between June and December, about one month (range 4 days-7 months) after the tick bite, the infection may cause heart complications known as Lyme carditis. Symptoms may include heart palpitations (in 69% of people), dizziness, fainting, shortness of breath, and chest pain. Other symptoms of Lyme disease may also be present, such as EM rash, joint aches, facial palsy, headaches, or radicular pain. In some people, however, carditis may be the first manifestation of Lyme disease. Lyme carditis in 19-87% of people adversely impacts the heart's electrical conduction system, causing atrioventricular block that often manifests as heart rhythms that alternate within minutes between abnormally slow and abnormally fast. In 10-15% of people, Lyme causes myocardial complications such as cardiomegaly, left ventricular dysfunction, or congestive heart failure.

Another skin condition, found in Europe but not in North America, is borrelial lymphocytoma, a purplish lump that develops on the ear lobe, nipple, or scrotum.

Late Disseminated Infection

After several months, untreated or inadequately treated people may go on to develop chronic symptoms that affect many parts of the body, including the joints, nerves, brain, eyes, and heart.

Lyme arthritis occurs in up to 60% of untreated people, typically starting about six months after infection. It usually affects only one or a few joints, often a knee or possibly the hip, other large joints, or the temporomandibular joint. There is usually large joint effusion and swelling, but only mild or moderate pain. Without treatment, swelling and pain typically resolve over time but periodically return. Baker's cysts may form and rupture. In some cases, joint erosion occurs.

Chronic neurologic symptoms occur in up to 5% of untreated people. A peripheral neuropathy or polyneuropathy may develop, causing abnormal sensations such as numbness, tingling or burning starting at the feet or hands and over time possibly moving up the limbs. A test may show reduced sensation of vibrations in the feet. An affected person may feel as if wearing a stocking or glove without actually doing so.

A neurologic syndrome called Lyme encephalopathy is associated with subtle memory and cognitive difficulties, insomnia, a general sense of feeling unwell, and changes in personality. However, problems such as depression and fibromyalgia are as common in people with Lyme disease as in the general population.

Lyme can cause a chronic encephalomyelitis that resembles multiple sclerosis. It may be progressive and can involve cognitive impairment, brain fog, migraines, balance issues, weakness in the legs, awkward gait, facial palsy, bladder problems, vertigo, and back pain. In rare cases, untreated Lyme disease may cause frank psychosis, which has been misdiagnosed as schizophrenia or bipolar disorder. Panic attacks and anxiety can occur; also, delusional behavior may be seen, including somatoform delusions, sometimes accompanied by a depersonalization or derealization syndrome, where the people begin to feel detached from themselves or from reality.

Acrodermatitis chronica atrophicans (ACA) is a chronic skin disorder observed primarily in Europe among the elderly. ACA begins as a reddish-blue patch of discolored skin, often on the backs of the hands or feet. The lesion slowly atrophies over several weeks or months, with the skin becoming first thin and wrinkled and then, if untreated, completely dry and hairless.

Cause

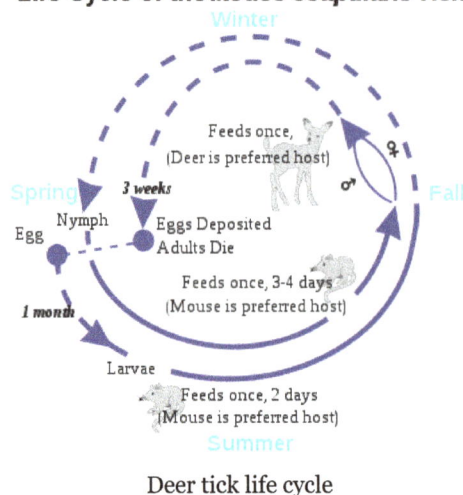

Deer tick life cycle

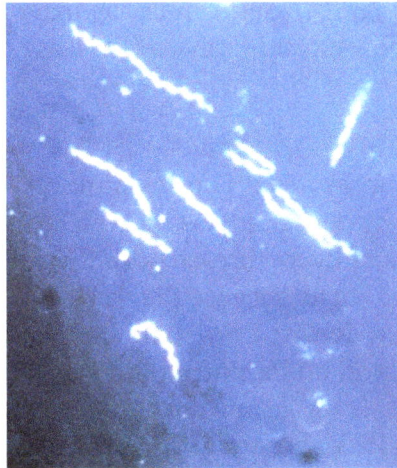

Borrelia bacteria, the causative agent of Lyme disease, magnified

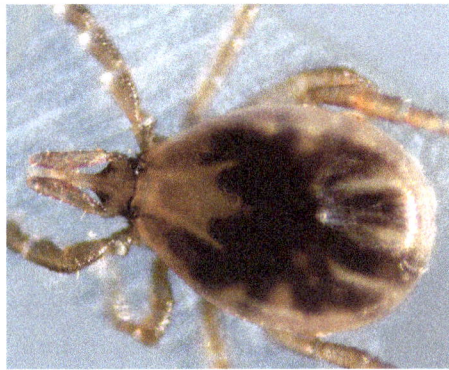

Ixodes scapularis, the primary vector of Lyme disease in eastern North America

Lyme disease is caused by spirochetes, spiral bacteria from the genus *Borrelia*. Spirochetes are surrounded by peptidoglycan and flagella, along with an outer membrane similar to other Gram-negative bacteria. Because of their double-membrane envelope, *Borrelia* bacteria are often mistakenly described as Gram negative despite the considerable differences in their envelope components from Gram-negative bacteria. The Lyme-related *Borrelia* species are collectively known as *Borrelia burgdorferi sensu lato*, and show a great deal of genetic diversity.

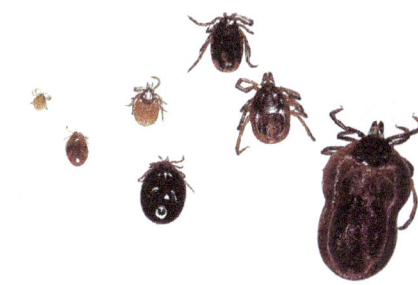

Tick *Ixodes ricinus*, developmental stages

B. burgdorferi sensu lato is made up of 21 closely related species, but only four clearly cause Lyme disease: *B. mayonii* (found in North America), *B. burgdorferi sensu stricto* (predominant in North America, but also present in Europe), *B. afzelii*, and *B. garinii* (both predominant in Eurasia).

Some studies have also proposed that *B. bissettii* and *B. valaisiana* may sometimes infect humans, but these species do not seem to be important causes of disease.

Transmission

Lyme disease is classified as a zoonosis, as it is transmitted to humans from a natural reservoir among small mammals and birds by ticks that feed on both sets of hosts. Hard-bodied ticks of the genus *Ixodes* are the main vectors of Lyme disease (also the vector for *Babesia*). Most infections are caused by ticks in the nymphal stage, because they are very small and thus may feed for long periods of time undetected. In New Jersey, USA, nymphal ticks are generally the size of a poppy seed and sometimes with a dark head and a translucent body. (The younger larval ticks are very rarely infected.) Although deer are the preferred hosts of adult deer ticks, and tick populations are much lower in the absence of deer, ticks generally do not acquire *Borrelia* from deer, instead they obtain them from infected small mammals such as the white-footed mouse, and occasionally birds. Areas where Lyme is common are expanding.

Within the tick midgut, the *Borrelia*'s outer surface protein A (OspA) binds to the tick receptor for OspA, known as TROSPA. When the tick feeds, the *Borrelia* downregulates OspA and upregulates OspC, another surface protein. After the bacteria migrate from the midgut to the salivary glands, OspC binds to Salp15, a tick salivary protein that appears to have immunosuppressive effects that enhance infection. Successful infection of the mammalian host depends on bacterial expression of OspC.

Tick bites often go unnoticed because of the small size of the tick in its nymphal stage, as well as tick secretions that prevent the host from feeling any itch or pain from the bite. However, transmission is quite rare, with only about 1% of recognized tick bites resulting in Lyme disease.

In Europe, the vector is *Ixodes ricinus*, which is also called the sheep tick or castor bean tick. In China, *Ixodes persulcatus* (the taiga tick) is probably the most important vector. In North America, the black-legged tick or deer tick (*Ixodes scapularis*) is the main vector on the East Coast.

The lone star tick (*Amblyomma americanum*), which is found throughout the Southeastern United States as far west as Texas, is unlikely to transmit the Lyme disease spirochetes, though it may be implicated in a related syndrome called southern tick-associated rash illness, which resembles a mild form of Lyme disease.

On the West Coast of the United States, the main vector is the western black-legged tick (*Ixodes pacificus*). The tendency of this tick species to feed predominantly on host species such as lizards that are resistant to *Borrelia* infection appears to diminish transmission of Lyme disease in the West.

Transmission can occur across the placenta during pregnancy and as with a number of other spirochetal diseases, adverse pregnancy outcomes are possible with untreated infection; prompt treatment with antibiotics reduces or eliminates this risk.

While Lyme spirochetes have been found in insects, as well as ticks, reports of actual infectious transmission appear to be rare. Lyme spirochete DNA has been found in semen and breast milk. However, according to the CDC, live spirochetes have not been found in breast milk, urine, or semen and thus is not sexually transmitted.

Tick-borne Coinfections

Ticks that transmit *B. burgdorferi* to humans can also carry and transmit several other parasites, such as *Theileria microti* and *Anaplasma phagocytophilum*, which cause the diseases babesiosis and human granulocytic anaplasmosis (HGA), respectively. Among people with early Lyme disease, depending on their location, 2–12% will also have HGA and 2–40% will have babesiosis. Ticks in certain regions, including the lands along the eastern Baltic Sea, also transmit tick-borne encephalitis.

Coinfections complicate Lyme symptoms, especially diagnosis and treatment. It is possible for a tick to carry and transmit one of the coinfections and not *Borrelia*, making diagnosis difficult and often elusive. The Centers for Disease Control and Prevention studied 100 ticks in rural New Jersey, and found 55% of the ticks were infected with at least one of the pathogens.

Pathophysiology

B. burgdorferi can spread throughout the body during the course of the disease, and has been found in the skin, heart, joints, peripheral nervous system, and central nervous system. Many of the signs and symptoms of Lyme disease are a consequence of the immune response to the spirochete in those tissues.

B. burgdorferi is injected into the skin by the bite of an infected *Ixodes* tick. Tick saliva, which accompanies the spirochete into the skin during the feeding process, contains substances that disrupt the immune response at the site of the bite. This provides a protective environment where the spirochete can establish infection. The spirochetes multiply and migrate outward within the dermis. The host inflammatory response to the bacteria in the skin causes the characteristic circular EM lesion. Neutrophils, however, which are necessary to eliminate the spirochetes from the skin, fail to appear in the developing EM lesion. This allows the bacteria to survive and eventually spread throughout the body.

Days to weeks following the tick bite, the spirochetes spread via the bloodstream to joints, heart, nervous system, and distant skin sites, where their presence gives rise to the variety of symptoms of the disseminated disease. The spread of *B. burgdorferi* is aided by the attachment of the host protease plasmin to the surface of the spirochete.

If untreated, the bacteria may persist in the body for months or even years, despite the production of *B. burgdorferi* antibodies by the immune system. The spirochetes may avoid the immune response by decreasing expression of surface proteins that are targeted by antibodies, antigenic variation of the VlsE surface protein, inactivating key immune components such as complement, and hiding in the extracellular matrix, which may interfere with the function of immune factors.

In the brain, *B. burgdorferi* may induce astrocytes to undergo astrogliosis (proliferation followed by apoptosis), which may contribute to neurodysfunction. The spirochetes may also induce host cells to secrete quinolinic acid, which stimulates the NMDA receptor on nerve cells, which may account for the fatigue and malaise observed with Lyme encephalopathy. In addition, diffuse white matter pathology during Lyme encephalopathy may disrupt gray matter connections, and could account for deficits in attention, memory, visuospatial ability, complex cognition, and emotional status. White matter disease may have a greater potential for recovery than gray matter disease, perhaps because the neuronal loss is less common. Resolution of MRI white matter hyperintensi-ties after antibiotic treatment has been observed.

Tryptophan, a precursor to serotonin, appears to be reduced within the central nervous system in a number of infectious diseases that affect the brain, including Lyme. Researchers are investigat-ing if this neurohormone secretion is the cause of neuropsychiatric disorders developing in some people with borreliosis.

Immunological Studies

Exposure to the *Borrelia* bacterium during Lyme disease possibly causes a long-lived and damag-ing inflammatory response, a form of pathogen-induced autoimmune disease. The production of this reaction might be due to a form of molecular mimicry, where *Borrelia* avoids being killed by the immune system by resembling normal parts of the body's tissues.

Chronic symptoms from an autoimmune reaction could explain why some symptoms persist even after the spirochetes have been eliminated from the body. This hypothesis may explain why chron-ic arthritis persists after antibiotic therapy, similar to rheumatic fever, but its wider application is controversial.

Diagnosis

Lyme disease is diagnosed based on symptoms, objective physical findings (such as erythema migrans (EM) rash, facial palsy, or arthritis), history of possible exposure to infected ticks, and possibly laboratory tests. People with symptoms of early Lyme disease should have a total body skin examination for EM rashes and be inquired if there was one in the past 1–2 months. Presence of an EM rash and recent tick exposure (i.e., being outdoors in a likely tick habitat where Lyme is common, within 30 days of the appearance of the rash) are sufficient for Lyme diagnosis; no laboratory confirmation is needed or recommended. Most people who get infect-ed do not remember a tick or a bite, and the EM rash need not look like a bull's eye (most EM rashes in the U.S. do not) or be accompanied by any other symptoms. In the U.S., Lyme is most common in the New England and Mid-Atlantic states and parts of Wisconsin and Minnesota, but it is expanding into other areas. Several bordering areas of Canada also offer high Lyme risk.

In the absence of an EM rash or history of tick exposure, Lyme diagnosis depends on laboratory confirmation. The bacteria that cause Lyme disease are difficult to observe directly in body tissues and also difficult and too time-consuming to grow in the laboratory. The most widely used tests look instead for presence of antibodies against those bacteria in the blood. A positive antibody test result does not by itself prove active infection, but can confirm an infection that is suspect-ed because of symptoms, objective findings, and history of tick exposure in a person. Because as many as 5-20% of the normal population have antibodies against Lyme, people without history and symptoms suggestive of Lyme disease should not be tested for Lyme antibodies: a positive result would likely be false, possibly causing unnecessary treatment.

In some cases, when history, signs, and symptoms are strongly suggestive of early disseminated Lyme disease, empiric treatment may be started and reevaluated as laboratory test results become available.

Laboratory Testing

Tests for antibodies in the blood by ELISA and Western blot is the most widely used method for Lyme diagnosis. A two-tiered protocol is recommended by the Centers for Disease Control and Prevention (CDC): the sensitive ELISA test is performed first, and if it is positive or equivocal, then the more specific Western blot is run. The immune system takes some time to produce antibodies in quantity. After Lyme infection onset, antibodies of types IgM and IgG usually can first be detected respectively at 2–4 weeks and 4–6 weeks, and peak at 6–8 weeks. When an EM rash first appears, antibodies usually cannot yet be detected; therefore, antibody confirmation at that time has no diagnostic value and is not recommended. Up to 30 days after suspected Lyme infection onset, infection can be confirmed by detection of IgM or IgG antibodies; after that, it is recommended that only IgG antibodies be considered. A positive IgM and negative IgG test result suggests an early infection, especially if confirmed several weeks later by a positive IgG test result. The number of IgM antibodies usually collapses 4–6 months after infection, while IgG antibodies can remain detectable for years. After antibiotic treatment, antibody tests become less useful. People treated when they have an EM rash often subsequently test negative for Lyme antibodies, whether treatment was successful or instead Lyme goes on to cause further complications. People treated later usually test positive before and after treatment, regardless of treatment success or failure. Better diagnostic tests are needed.

The reliability of the CDC two-tiered protocol is controversial. Studies show the Western blot IgM has a specificity of 94–96% for people with clinical symptoms of early Lyme disease. The initial ELISA test has a sensitivity of about 70%, and in two-tiered testing, the overall sensitivity is only 64%, although this rises to 100% in the subset of people with disseminated symptoms, such as arthritis. Erroneous test results have been widely reported in both early and late stages of the disease, and can be caused by several factors, including antibody cross-reactions from other infections, including Epstein–Barr virus and cytomegalovirus, as well as herpes simplex virus. The overall rate of false positives is low, only about 1 to 3%, in comparison to a false-negative rate of up to 36% in the early stages of infection using two-tiered testing.

Other tests may be used in neuroborreliosis cases. In Europe, neuroborreliosis is usually caused by Borrelia garinii and almost always involves lymphocytic pleocytosis, i.e. the densities of lymphocytes (infection-fighting cells) and protein in the cerebrospinal fluid (CSF) typically rise to characteristically abnormal levels, while glucose level remains normal. Additionally, the immune system produces antibodies against Lyme inside the intrathecal space, which contains the CSF. Demonstration by lumbar puncture and CSF analysis of pleocytosis and intrathecal antibody production are required for definite diagnosis of neuroborreliosis in Europe (except in cases of peripheral neuropathy associated with acrodermatitis chronica atrophicans, which usually is caused by Borrelia afzelii and confirmed by blood antibody tests). In North America, neuroborreliosis is caused by Borrelia burgdorferi and may not be accompanied by the same CSF signs; they confirm a diagnosis of central nervous system (CNS) neuroborreliosis if positive, but do not exclude it if negative. American guidelines consider CSF analysis optional when symptoms appear to be confined to the peripheral nervous system (PNS), e.g. facial palsy without overt meninigitis symptoms. Unlike blood and intrathecal antibody tests, CSF pleocytosis tests revert to normal after infection ends and therefore can be used as objective markers of treatment success and inform decisions on whether to retreat. In infection involving the PNS, electromyography and nerve conduction studies can be used to monitor objectively the response to treatment.

In Lyme carditis, electrocardiograms are used to evidence heart conduction abnormalities, while echocardiography may show myocardial dysfunction. Biopsy and confirmation of Borrelia cells in myocardial tissue may be used in specific cases but are usually not done because of risk of the procedure.

Polymerase chain reaction (PCR) tests for Lyme disease have also been developed to detect the genetic material (DNA) of the Lyme disease spirochete. Culture or PCR are the current means for detecting the presence of the organism, as serologic studies only test for antibodies of *Borrelia*. PCR has the advantage of being much faster than culture. However, PCR tests are susceptible to false positive results, e.g. by detection of debris of dead Borrelia cells or specimen contamination. Even when properly performed, PCR often shows false negative results because few Borrelia cells can be found in blood and cerebrospinal fluid (CSF) during infection. Hence, PCR tests are recommended only in special cases, e.g. diagnosis of Lyme arthritis, because it is a highly sensitive way of detecting *ospA* DNA in synovial fluid. Although sensitivity of PCR in CSF is low, its use may be considered when intrathecal antibody production test results are suspected of being falsely negative, e.g. in very early (< 6 weeks) neuroborreliosis or in immunosuppressed people.

Several other forms of laboratory testing for Lyme disease are available, some of which have not been adequately validated. OspA antigens, shed by live *Borrelia* bacteria into urine, are a promising technique being studied. The use of nanotrap particles for their detection is being looked at and the OspA has been linked to active symptoms of Lyme. High titers of either immunoglobulin G (IgG) or immunoglobulin M (IgM) antibodies to *Borrelia* antigens indicate disease, but lower titers can be misleading, because the IgM antibodies may remain after the initial infection, and IgG antibodies may remain for years.

The CDC does not recommend urine antigen tests, PCR tests on urine, immunofluorescent staining for cell-wall-deficient forms of *B. burgdorferi*, and lymphocyte transformation tests.

Imaging

Neuroimaging is controversial in whether it provides specific patterns unique to neuroborreliosis, but may aid in differential diagnosis and in understanding the pathophysiology of the disease. Though controversial, some evidence shows certain neuroimaging tests can provide data that are helpful in the diagnosis of a person. Magnetic resonance imaging (MRI) and single-photon emission computed tomography (SPECT) are two of the tests that can identify abnormalities in the brain of a person affected with this disease. Neuroimaging findings in an MRI include lesions in the periventricular white matter, as well as enlarged ventricles and cortical atrophy. The findings are considered somewhat unexceptional because the lesions have been found to be reversible following antibiotic treatment. Images produced using SPECT show numerous areas where an insufficient amount of blood is being delivered to the cortex and subcortical white matter. However, SPECT images are known to be nonspecific because they show a heterogeneous pattern in the imaging. The abnormalities seen in the SPECT images are very similar to those seen in people with cerebral vacuities and Creutzfeldt–Jakob disease, which makes them questionable.

Differential Diagnosis

Community clinics have been reported to misdiagnose 23-28% of Erythema migrans (EM) rashes and 83% of other objective manifestations of early Lyme disease. EM rashes are often misdiagnosed as spider bites, cellulitis, or shingles. Many misdiagnoses are credited to the widespread misconception that EM rashes should look like a bull's eye. Actually, the key distinguishing features of the EM rash are the speed and extent to which it expands, respectively up to 2–3 cm/day and a diameter of at least 5 cm, and in 50% of cases more than 16 cm. The rash expands away from its center, which may or may not look different or be separated by ring-like clearing from the rest of the rash. Compared to EM rashes, spider bites are more common in the limbs, tend to be more painful and itchy or become swollen, and some may cause necrosis (sinking dark blue patch of dead skin). Cellulitis most commonly develops around a wound or ulcer, is rarely circular, and is more likely to become swollen and tender. EM rashes often appear at sites that are unusual for cellulitis, such as the armpit, groin, abdomen, or back of knee. Like Lyme, shingles often begins with headache, fever, and fatigue, which are followed by pain or numbness. However, unlike Lyme, in shingles these symptoms are usually followed by appearance of rashes composed of multiple small blisters along a nerve's dermatome, and shingles can also be confirmed by quick laboratory tests.

Facial palsy caused by Lyme disease (LDFP) is often misdiagnosed as Bell's palsy. Although Bell's palsy is the most common type of one-sided facial palsy (about 70% of cases), LDFP can account for about 25% of cases of facial palsy in areas where Lyme disease is common. Compared to LDFP, Bell's palsy much less frequently affects both sides of the face. Even though LDFP and Bell's palsy have similar symptoms and evolve similarly if untreated, corticosteroid treatment is beneficial for Bell's Palsy, while being detrimental for LDFP. Recent history of exposure to a likely tick habitat during warmer months, EM rash, viral-like symptoms such as headache and fever, and/or palsy in both sides of the face should be evaluated for likelihood of LDFP; if it is more than minimal, empiric therapy with antibiotics should be initiated, without corticosteroids, and reevaluated upon completion of laboratory tests for Lyme disease.

Unlike viral meningitis, Lyme lymphocytic meningitis tends to not cause fever, last longer, and recur. Lymphocytic meningitis is also characterized by possibly co-occurring with EM rash, facial palsy, or partial vision obstruction and having much lower percentage of polymorphonuclear leukocytes in CSF.

Lyme radiculopathy affecting the limbs is often misdiagnosed as a radiculopathy caused by nerve root compression, such as sciatica. Although most cases of radiculopathy are compressive and resolve with conservative treatment (e.g., rest) within 4–6 weeks, guidelines for managing radiculopathy recommend first evaluating risks of other possible causes that, although less frequent, require immediate diagnosis and treatment, including infections such as Lyme and shingles. A history of outdoor activities in likely tick habitats in the last 3 months possibly followed by a rash or viral-like symptoms, and current headache, other symptoms of lymphocytic meningitis, or facial palsy would lead to suspicion of Lyme disease and recommendation of serological and lumbar puncture tests for confirmation.

Lyme radiculopathy affecting the trunk can be misdiagnosed as myriad other conditions, such as diverticulitis and acute coronary syndrome. Diagnosis of late-stage Lyme disease is often complicated by a multifaceted appearance and nonspecific symptoms, prompting one reviewer to call

Lyme the new "great imitator". Lyme disease may be misdiagnosed as multiple sclerosis, rheumatoid arthritis, fibromyalgia, chronic fatigue syndrome, lupus, Crohn's disease, HIV, or other autoimmune and neurodegenerative diseases. As all people with later-stage infection will have a positive antibody test, simple blood tests can exclude Lyme disease as a possible cause of a person's symptoms.

Prevention

Tick bites may be prevented by avoiding or reducing time in likely tick habitats and taking precautions while in and when getting out of one.

Most Lyme human infections are caused by Ixodes nymph bites between April and September. Ticks prefer moist, shaded locations in woodlands, shrubs, tall grasses and leaf litter or wood piles. Tick densities tend to be highest in woodlands, followed by unmaintained edges between woods and lawns (about half as high), ornamental plants and perennial groundcover (about a quarter), and lawns (about 30 times less). Ixodes larvae and nymphs tend to be abundant also where mice nest, such as stone walls and wood logs. Ixodes larvae and nymphs typically wait for potential hosts ("quest") on leaves or grasses close to the ground with forelegs outstretched; when a host brushes against its limbs, the tick rapidly clings and climbs on the host looking for a skin location to bite. In Northeastern United States, 69% of tick bites are estimated to happen in residences, 11% in schools or camps, 9% in parks or recreational areas, 4% at work, 3% while hunting, and 4% in other areas. Activities associated with tick bites around residences include yard work, brush clearing, gardening, playing in the yard, and letting into the house dogs or cats that roam outside in woody or grassy areas. In parks, tick bites often happen while hiking or camping. Walking on a mowed lawn or center of a trail without touching adjacent vegetation is less risky than crawling or sitting on a log or stone wall. Pets should not be allowed to roam freely in likely tick habitats.

As a precaution, CDC recommends soaking or spraying clothes, shoes, and camping gear such as tents, backpacks and sleeping bags with 0.5% permethrin solution and hanging them to dry before use. Permethrin is odorless and safe for humans but highly toxic to ticks. After crawling on permethrin-treated fabric for as few as 10–20 seconds, tick nymphs become irritated and fall off or die. Permethrin-treated closed-toed shoes and socks reduce by 74 times the number of bites from nymphs that make first contact with a shoe of a person also wearing treated shorts (because nymphs usually quest near the ground, this is a typical contact scenario). Better protection can be achieved by tucking permethrin-treated trousers (pants) into treated socks and a treated long-sleeve shirt into the trousers so as to minimize gaps through which a tick might reach the wearer's skin. Light-colored clothing may make it easier to see ticks and remove them before they bite. Military and outdoor workers' uniforms treated with permethrin have been found to reduce the number of bite cases by 80-95%. Permethrin protection lasts several weeks of wear and washings in customer-treated items and up to 70 washings for factory-treated items. Permethrin should not be used on human skin, underwear or cats.

The EPA recommends several tick repellents for use on exposed skin, including DEET, picaridin, IR3535 (a derivative of amino acid beta-alanine), oil of lemon eucalyptus (OLE, a natural compound) and OLE's active ingredient para-menthane-diol (PMD). Unlike permethrin, repellents repel but do not kill ticks, protect for only several hours after application, and may be washed off by sweat or water. The most popular repellent is DEET in the U.S. and picaridin in Europe.

Unlike DEET, picaridin is odorless and is less likely to irritate the skin or harm fabric or plastics. Repellents with higher concentration may last longer but are not more effective; against ticks, 20% picaridin may work for 8 hours vs. 55-98.11% DEET for 5–6 hours or 30-40% OLE for 6 hours. Repellents should not be used under clothes, on eyes, mouth, wounds or cuts, or on babies younger than 2 months (3 years for OLE or PMD). If sunscreen is used, repellent should be applied on top of it. Repellents should not be sprayed directly on a face, but should instead be sprayed on a hand and then rubbed on the face.

After coming indoors, clothes, gear and pets should be checked for ticks. Clothes can be put into a hot dryer for 10 minutes to kill ticks (just washing or warm dryer are not enough). Showering as soon as possible, looking for ticks over the entire body, and removing them reduce risk of infection. Unfed tick nymphs are the size of a poppy seed, but a day or two after biting and attaching themselves to a person, they look like a small blood blister. The following areas should be checked especially carefully: armpits, between legs, back of knee, bellybutton, trunk, and in children ears, neck and hair.

Tick Removal

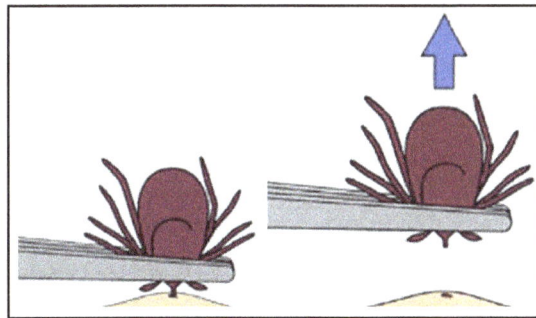

Removal of a tick using tweezers

Attached ticks should be removed promptly. Risk of infection increases with time of attachment, but in North America risk of Lyme disease is small if the tick is removed within 36 hours. CDC recommends inserting a fine-tipped tweezer between the skin and the tick, grasping very firmly, and pulling the closed tweezer straight away from the skin without twisting, jerking, squeezing or crushing the tick. After tick removal, any tick parts remaining in the skin should be removed with the tweezer, if possible. Wound and hands should then be cleaned with alcohol or soap and water. The tick may be disposed by placing it in a container with alcohol, sealed bag, tape or flushed down the toilet. The bitten person should write down where and when the bite happened so that this can be informed to a doctor if the person gets a rash or flu-like symptoms in the following several weeks. CDC recommends not using fingers, nail polish, petroleum jelly or heat on the tick to try to remove it.

In Australia, where the Australian paralysis tick is prevalent, the Australasian Society of Clinical Immunology and Allergy recommends not using tweezers to remove ticks, because if the person is allergic, anaphylaxis could result. Instead, a product should be sprayed on the tick to cause it to freeze and then drop off. A doctor would use liquid nitrogen, but products available from drugstores for freezing warts can be used instead. Another method originating from Australia consists in using about 20 cm of dental floss or fishing line for slowly tying an overhand knot between the skin and the tick and then pulling it away from the skin.

Preventive Antibiotics

The risk of infectious transmission increases with the duration of tick attachment. It requires between 36 and 48 hours of attachment for the bacteria that causes Lyme to travel from within the tick into its saliva. If a deer tick that is sufficiently likely to be carrying *Borrelia* is found attached to a person and removed, and if the tick has been attached for 36 hours or is engorged, a single dose of doxycycline administered within the 72 hours after removal may reduce the risk of Lyme disease. It is not generally recommended for all people bitten, as development of infection is rare: about 50 bitten people would have to be treated this way to prevent one case of erythema migrans (i.e. the typical rash found in about 70-80% of people infected).

Garden Landscaping

Several landscaping practices may reduce risk of tick bites in residential yards. The lawn should be kept mowed, leaf litter and weeds removed and groundcover use avoided. Woodlands, shrubs, stone walls and wood piles should be separated from the lawn by a 3-ft-wide rock or woodchip barrier. Without vegetation on the barrier, ticks will tend not to cross it; acaricides may also be sprayed on it to kill ticks. A sun-exposed tick-safe zone at least 9 ft from the barrier should concentrate human activity on the yard, including any patios, playgrounds and gardening. Materials such as wood decking, concrete, bricks, gravel or woodchips may be used on the ground under patios and playgrounds so as to discourage ticks there. An 8-ft-high fence may be added to keep deer away from the tick-safe zone.

Occupational Exposure

Outdoor workers are at risk of Lyme disease if they work at sites with infected ticks. This includes construction, landscaping, forestry, brush clearing, land surveying, farming, railroad work, oil field work, utility line work, park or wildlife management. U.S. workers in the northeastern and north-central states are at highest risk of exposure to infected ticks. Ticks may also transmit other tick-borne diseases to workers in these and other regions of the country. Worksites with woods, bushes, high grass or leaf litter are likely to have more ticks. Outdoor workers should be most careful to protect themselves in the late spring and summer when young ticks are most active.

Host Animals

Lyme and other deer tick-borne diseases can sometimes be reduced by greatly reducing the deer population on which the adult ticks depend for feeding and reproduction. Lyme disease cases fell following deer eradication on an island, Monhegan, Maine and following deer control in Mumford Cove, Connecticut. It is worth noting that eliminating deer may lead to a temporary increase in tick density.

For example, in the U.S., reducing the deer population to levels of 8 to 10 per square mile (from the current levels of 60 or more deer per square mile in the areas of the country with the highest Lyme disease rates) may reduce tick numbers and reduce the spread of Lyme and other tick-borne diseases. However, such a drastic reduction may be very difficult to implement in many areas, and low to moderate densities of deer or other large mammal hosts may continue to feed sufficient adult ticks to maintain larval densities at high levels. Routine veterinary control of ticks of domestic animals, including livestock, by use of acaricides can contribute to reducing exposure of humans to ticks.

In Europe, known reservoirs of *Borrelia burgdorferi* were 9 small mammals, 7 medium-sized mammals and 16 species of birds (including passerines, sea-birds and pheasants). These animals seem to transmit spirochetes to ticks and thus participate in the natural circulation of B. burgdorferi in Europe. The house mouse is also suspected as well as other species of small rodents, particularly in Eastern Europe and Russia. "The reservoir species that contain the most pathogens are the European roe deer *Capreolus capreolus*; "*it does not appear to serve as a major reservoir of B. burgdorferi*" thought Jaenson & al. (incompetent host for *B. burgdorferi* and TBE virus) but it is important for feeding the ticks, as red deer and wild boars (*Sus scrofa*), in which one *Rickettsia* and three *Borrelia* species were identified", with high risks of coinfection in roe deer. Nevertheless, in the 2000s, in roe deer in Europe "*two species of Rickettsia and two species of Borrelia were identified*".

Vaccination

A recombinant vaccine against Lyme disease, based on the outer surface protein A (ospA) of *B. burgdorferi*, was developed by SmithKline Beecham. In clinical trials involving more than 10,000 people, the vaccine, called LYMErix, was found to confer protective immunity to *Borrelia* in 76% of adults and 100% of children with only mild or moderate and transient adverse effects. LYMErix was approved on the basis of these trials by the Food and Drug Administration (FDA) on 21 December 1998.

Following approval of the vaccine, its entry in clinical practice was slow for a variety of reasons, including its cost, which was often not reimbursed by insurance companies. Subsequently, hundreds of vaccine recipients reported they had developed autoimmune and other side effects. Supported by some advocacy groups, a number of class-action lawsuits were filed against GlaxoSmithKline, alleging the vaccine had caused these health problems. These claims were investigated by the FDA and the Centers for Disease Control, which found no connection between the vaccine and the autoimmune complaints.

Despite the lack of evidence that the complaints were caused by the vaccine, sales plummeted and LYMErix was withdrawn from the U.S. market by GlaxoSmithKline in February 2002, in the setting of negative media coverage and fears of vaccine side effects. The fate of LYMErix was described in the medical literature as a "cautionary tale"; an editorial in *Nature* cited the withdrawal of LYMErix as an instance in which "unfounded public fears place pressures on vaccine developers that go beyond reasonable safety considerations." The original developer of the OspA vaccine at the Max Planck Institute told *Nature*: "This just shows how irrational the world can be. There was no scientific justification for the first OspA vaccine LYMErix being pulled."

Vaccines have been formulated and approved for prevention of Lyme disease in dogs. Currently, three Lyme disease vaccines are available. LymeVax, formulated by Fort Dodge Laboratories, contains intact dead spirochetes which expose the host to the organism. Galaxy Lyme, Intervet-Schering-Plough's vaccine, targets proteins OspC and OspA. The OspC antibodies kill any of the bacteria that have not been killed by the OspA antibodies. Canine Recombinant Lyme, formulated by Merial, generates antibodies against the OspA protein so a tick feeding on a vaccinated dog draws in blood full of anti-OspA antibodies, which kill the spirochetes in the tick's gut before they are transmitted to the dog.

A hexavalent (OspA) protein subunit-based vaccine candidate VLA15 was granted fast track designation by the U.S. Food and Drug Administration in 2017 which will allow further study.

Treatment

Antibiotics are the primary treatment. The specific approach to their use is dependent on the individual affected and the stage of the disease. For most people with early localized infection, oral administration of doxycycline is widely recommended as the first choice, as it is effective against not only *Borrelia* bacteria but also a variety of other illnesses carried by ticks. People taking doxycycline should avoid sun exposure because of higher risk of sunburns. Doxycycline is contraindicated in children younger than eight years of age and women who are pregnant or breastfeeding; alternatives to doxycycline are amoxicillin, cefuroxime axetil, and azithromycin. Azithromicyn is recommended only in case of intolerance to the other antibiotics. The standard treatment for cellulitis, cephalexin, is not useful for Lyme disease. When it is unclear if a rash is caused by Lyme or cellulitis, the IDSA recommends treatment with cefuroxime or amoxicillin/clavulanic acid, as these are effective against both infections. Individuals with early disseminated or late Lyme infection may have symptomatic cardiac disease, Lyme arthritis, or neurologic symptoms like facial palsy, radiculopathy, meningitis, or peripheral neuropathy. Intravenous administration of ceftriaxone is recommended as the first choice in these cases; cefotaxime and doxycycline are available as alternatives.

These treatment regimens last from one to four weeks. Neurologic complications of Lyme disease may be treated with doxycycline as it can be taken by mouth and has a lower cost, although in North America evidence of efficacy is only indirect. In case of failure, guidelines recommend retreatment with injectable ceftriaxone. Several months after treatment for Lyme arthritis, if joint swelling persists or returns, a second round of antibiotics may be considered; intravenous antibiotics are preferred for retreatment in case of poor response to oral antibiotics. Outside of that, a prolonged antibiotic regimen lasting more than 28 days is not recommended as no evidence shows it to be effective. IgM and IgG antibody levels may be elevated for years even after successful treatment with antibiotics. As antibody levels are not indicative of treatment success, testing for them is not recommended.

Facial palsy may resolve without treatment, however, antibiotic treatment is recommended to stop other Lyme complications. Corticosteroids are not recommended when facial palsy is caused by Lyme disease. In those with facial palsy, frequent use of artificial tears while awake is recommended, along with ointment and a patch or taping the eye closed when sleeping.

About a third of people with Lyme carditis need a temporary pacemaker until their heart conduction abnormality resolves, and 21% need to be hospitalized. Lyme carditis should not be treated with corticosteroids.

People with Lyme arthritis should limit their level of physical activity to avoid damaging affected joints, and in case of limping should use crutches. Pain associated with Lyme disease may be treated with nonsteroidal anti-inflammatory drugs (NSAIDs). Corticosteroid joint injections are not recommended for Lyme arthritis that is being treated with antibiotics. People with Lyme arthritis treated with intravenous antibiotics or two months of oral antibiotics who continue to have joint swelling two months after treatment and have negative PCR test for Borrelia DNA in the synovial fluid are said to have antibiotic-refractory Lyme arthritis; this is more common after infection by certain Borrelia strains in people with certain genetic and immunologic characteristics. Antibiotic-refractory Lyme arthritis may be symptomatically treated with NSAIDs, disease-modifying antirheumatic drugs (DMARDs), or arthroscopic synovectomy. Physical therapy is recommended for adults after resolution of Lyme arthritis.

People receiving treatment should be advised that reinfection is possible and how to prevent it.

Prognosis

Lyme disease's typical first sign, the erythema migrans (EM) rash, resolves within several weeks even without treatment. However, in untreated people, the infection often disseminates to the nervous system, heart, or joints, possibly causing permanent damage to body tissues.

People who receive recommended antibiotic treatment within several days of appearance of an initial EM rash have the best prospects. Recovery may not be total or immediate. The percentage of people achieving full recovery in the United States increases from about 64-71% at end of treatment for EM rash to about 84-90% after 30 months; higher percentages are reported in Europe. Treatment failure, i.e. persistence of original or appearance of new signs of the disease, occurs only in a few people. Remaining people are considered cured but continue to experience subjective symptoms, e.g. joint or muscle pains or fatigue. These symptoms usually are mild and nondisabling.

People treated only after nervous system manifestations of the disease may end up with objective neurological deficits, in addition to subjective symptoms. In Europe, an average of 32–33 months after initial Lyme symptoms in people treated mostly with doxycycline 200 mg for 14–21 days, the percentage of people with lingering symptoms was much higher among those diagnosed with neuroborreliosis (50%) than among those with only an EM rash (16%). In another European study, 5 years after treatment for neuroborreliosis, lingering symptoms were less common among children (15%) than adults (30%), and in the latter was less common among those treated within 30 days of the first symptom (16%) than among those treated later (39%); among those with lingering symptoms, 54% had daily activities restricted and 19% were on sick leave or incapacitated.

Some data suggest that about 90% of Lyme facial palsies treated with antibiotics recover fully a median of 24 days after appearing and most of the rest recover with only mild abnormality. However, in Europe 41% of people treated for facial palsy had other lingering symptoms at followup up to 6 months later, including 28% with numbness or altered sensation and 14% with fatigue or concentration problems. Palsies in both sides of the face are associated with worse and longer time to recovery. Historical data suggests that untreated people with facial palsies recover at nearly the same rate, but 88% subsequently have Lyme arthritis. Other research shows that synkinesis (involuntary movement of a facial muscle when another one is voluntarily moved) can become evident only 6–12 months after facial palsy appears to be resolved, as damaged nerves regrow and sometimes connect to incorrect muscles. Synkinesis is associated with corticosteroid use. In longer-term follow-up, 16-23% of Lyme facial palsies do not fully recover.

In Europe, about a quarter of people with Bannwarth syndrome (Lyme radiculopathy and lymphocytic meningitis) treated with intravenous ceftriaxone for 14 days an average of 30 days after first symptoms had to be retreated 3–6 months later because of unsatisfactory clinical response or continued objective markers of infection in cerebrospinal fluid; after 12 months, 64% recovered fully, 31% had nondisabling mild or infrequent symptoms that did not require regular use of analgesics, and 5% had symptoms that were disabling or required substantial use of analgesics. The most common lingering nondisabling symptoms were headache, fatigue, altered sensation, joint pains, memory disturbances, malaise, radicular pain, sleep disturbances, muscle pains, and concentration disturbances. Lingering disabling symptoms included facial palsy and other impaired movement.

Recovery from late neuroborreliosis tends to take longer and be less complete than from early neuroborreliosis, probably because of irreversible neurologic damage.

About half the people with Lyme carditis progress to complete heart block, but it usually resolves in a week. Other Lyme heart conduction abnormalities resolve typically within 6 weeks. About 94% of people have full recovery, but 5% need a permanent pacemaker and 1% end up with persistent heart block (the actual percentage may be higher because of unrecognized cases). Lyme myocardial complications usually are mild and self-limiting. However, in some cases Lyme carditis can be fatal.

Recommended antibiotic treatments are effective in about 90% of Lyme arthritis cases, although it can take several months for inflammation to resolve and a second round of antibiotics is often necessary. Antibiotic-refractory Lyme arthritis also eventually resolves, typically within 9–14 months (range 4 months-4 years); DMARDs or synovectomy can accelerate recovery.

Reinfection is not uncommon. In a U.S. study, 6-11% of people treated for an EM rash had another EM rash within 30 months. The second rash typically is due to infection by a different Borrelia strain.

People who have nonspecific, subjective symptoms such as fatigue, joint and muscle aches, or cognitive difficulties for more than six months after recommended treatment for Lyme disease are said to have post-treatment Lyme disease syndrome. As of 2016 the reason for the lingering symptoms was not known; the condition is generally managed similarly to fibromyalgia or chronic fatigue syndrome.

West Nile Virus

West Nile Virus (WNV) is a potentially life-threatening viral infection. It can pass to animals and humans if they are bitten by an infected mosquito. WNV is a virus of the Flaviviridae family, which includes the viruses responsible for Japanese encephalitis and dengue fever.

It mainly affects birds, but it can also be experienced by mammals and reptiles. Between 70 and 80 percent of people have no symptoms. Up to one percent of those who become ill have serious and potentially fatal complications.

West Nile Virus (WNV) used to exist only in temperate and tropical areas, but in 1999, infections appeared in New York. It has since spread across most of the United States (U.S.), and is a notifiable disease.

Signs and Symptoms

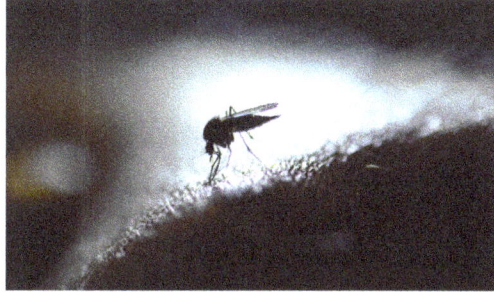

West Nile Virus is transferred to humans by mosquitos.
They pick up the virus from deceased birds

WNV can affect humans in three different ways:

- Asymptomatic infection: In about 80 percent of cases, there are no signs or symptoms.

- West Nile Fever: Around 20 percent of people experience a mild febrile syndrome.

- Neuroinvasive disease: About 1 percent of patients develop complications in the central nervous system (CNS) that affect the brain and spine.

West Nile Fever

Symptoms appear 2 to 8 days after infection. This is known as the incubation period.

They may include:

- Backache and muscle aches

- Fever and excessive sweating

- Diarrhea, nausea, vomiting, and loss of appetite

- Drowsiness

- Headache

- Skin rash

- Swollen lymph nodes, or glands.

These symptoms resolve within 7 to 10 days. Fatigue may linger for several weeks, while glands may be swollen for up to 2 months.

Neuroinvasive Disease

Around 1 percent of infected individuals develop more serious neurological infections, and around 10 percent of these cases are fatal.

Possible complications are:

- Encephalitis: Inflammation of the brain

- Meningitis: Inflammation of tissues surrounding the brain and spinal cord

- Myelitis, or West Nile poliomyelitis: Inflammation of the spinal cord

- Acute flaccid paralysis: Sudden weakness in the arms, legs and breathing muscles.

Signs and symptoms may include:

- Confusion and disorientation

- Convulsions

- High fever

- Muscle jerking

- Pain

- Parkinson's disease-like symptoms, including tremors

- Sudden weakness, poor coordination, and partial paralysis

- Severe headache

- Stiff neck

- Stupor

- Coma.

Most at risk are people aged over 60 years and those with existing conditions, such as kidney disease, diabetes, cancer, and conditions that weaken the immune system.

Some neurological effects can be permanent.

Causes and Risk Factors

Infected birds have high levels of the virus. In the U.S., the American robin and the American crow are common carriers. If a mosquito bites an infected bird, and it then bites a person, the virus will enter the bloodstream of that individual. The Culex Pipiens mosquito is known to pass on WNV in the U.S.

It remains unknown exactly how the virus works. WNV enters the bloodstream and reproduces, and sometimes it can cross the blood-brain barrier to cause inflammation in the brain.

Transmission is also possible through:

- Blood transfusions: Health authorities now screen patients for WNV before accepting a transfusion.

- Organ transplants: According to the Centers for Disease Control and Prevention, some centers test organ donors for WNV, whereas others do not.

- Pregnancy: An infected mother can infect her fetus, but the risk is very low.

- Breast-feeding: There is a very small chance of passing on the virus through breast milk, but the risk is so small that the Centers for Disease Control and Prevention (CDC) advise mothers to continue breast-feeding.

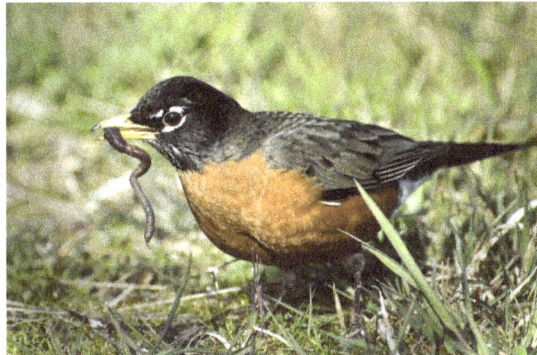

The American robin is one of the key culprits for the presence of WNV

Risk Factors

Certain factors increase the risk of infection:

- Seasons: In temperate areas, WNV begins to appear in early spring. Infections peak in late summer and early fall. In tropical and some sub-tropical areas, there is a year-round risk of infection.

- Location: Living in or visiting an area known to have WNV increases the risk of infection. In the U.S., this includes all states except Alaska and Hawaii.

- Exposure to mosquitoes: Spending more time outdoors increases the chance of infection after being bitten by an infected mosquito.

Laboratory work: Infection can occur in laboratories where WNV is present.

Diagnosis

The doctor will ask about symptoms and carry out a physical examination.

The following diagnostic tests may be ordered:

- Blood test: This may reveal higher-than-normal levels of antibodies to WNV. A complete blood count may be done.

- CT or MRI scan of the head: This can sometimes reveal brain inflammation and swelling.

- Lumbar puncture, or spinal tap: This can diagnose meningitis.

In a lumbar puncture, cerebrospinal fluid from around the brain and spinal cord is extracted. A needle is inserted between the lower vertebrae of the spine. A high level of white cells suggests an infection.

Treatment

Most patients make a full recovery without medical treatment. Over-the-counter (OTC) treatments can help with symptom relief.

Severe symptoms will require hospitalization and supportive treatment, such as assistance with breathing and intravenous fluids.

Prevention

There is currently no vaccine available to protect against WNV.

Humans cannot pass on the disease, so the best prevention is to avoid being bitten by mosquitoes.

Things to consider include:

- Clothing: Cover as much skin as possible. Wear long-sleeved shirts, long pants, high socks, and a hat. Some people tuck the bottom of their pants into their socks.

- Mosquito repellents: Use one with at least 10 percent concentration of DEET. DEET should not be used on young children, and insect repellent should not be used on infants under 2 months.

- Mosquito traps, nets, and screens: Maintain screens on doors and windows, and have nets over beds and children's strollers. Ensure that there are no holes.

- Smell: Avoid heavily scented soaps and perfumes, as these can attract mosquitoes.

- Camping: Treat clothes, shoes and camping gear beforehand with permethrin. Specially treated clothes are available from some stores.

- The time of day: Mosquitoes are more plentiful at dawn and dusk.

- Stagnant water: Mosquitoes breed in clean, stagnant water.

- To reduce the risk of WNV due to stagnant water.

- Check and remove stagnant water from around the home, and avoid camping near lakes and ponds.

- Turning over pails and watering cans and storing them under shelter can prevent them filling with water.

- Remove the water from plant pot plates, or avoid using them, if possible. Loosen hard soil from potted plants to prevent puddles from developing on the surface.

- Change the water in flower vases every two days, and scrub and rinse the inside of the vase thoroughly each time.

- Keep leaves from causing puddles.

To remove mosquito eggs, thoroughly clean and scrub pot plates, pails, and other containers. Keep scupper drains unblocked and do not cover them with plants or other items. Cover rarely used gully traps, use non-perforated traps, and install anti-mosquito valves. Do not place receptacles under or on top of air-conditioning units. Along with reporting any dead birds to the authorities, these measures can help to prevent WNV in the wider community.

References

- Decker, Janet (2003). Deadly Diseases and Epidemics, Anthrax. Chelesa House Publishers. pp. 27–28. ISBN 978-0-7910-7302-5

- Gajula V, Kamepalli R, Kalavakunta JK (2014). "A star in the eye: cat scratch neuroretinitis". Clinical Case Reports. 2 (1): 17. doi:10.1002/ccr3.43. PMC 4184768. PMID 25356231

- "Plague war: The 1979 anthrax leak". Frontline. PBS. Archived from the original on 17 September 2008. Retrieved 13 August, 2008

- Tordo, N; Bourhy, H; Sacramento, D (1994). "Ch. 10: PCR technology for lyssavirus diagnosis". In Clewley, J.P. (ed.). The Polymerase Chain Reaction (PCR) for Human Viral Diagnosis. CRC Press. pp. 125–145. ISBN 978-0-8493-4833-4.

- Gear JH, Ryan J, Rossouw E (February 1978). "A consideration of the diagnosis of dangerous infectious fevers in South Africa". South African Medical Journal. 53 (7): 235–37. PMID 565951

4
Veterinary Practices and Surgical Procedures

Veterinary surgery is broadly classified into three categories, soft-tissue surgery, orthopedics and neurosurgery. Some of the common surgical procedures which are conducted on animals are onychectomy, devocalization, docking, urethrostomy and triple tibial osteotomy. The chapter closely examines these surgical practices to provide an extensive understanding of the subject.

Onychectomy

Declawing is a series of bone amputations. Declawing is more accurately described by the term de-knuckling and is not merely the removal of the claws, as the term "declawing" implies. In humans, fingernails grow from the skin, but in animals that hunt prey, the claws grow from the bone; therefore, the last bone is amputated so the claw cannot re-grow. The last bone of each of the ten front toes of a cat's paw is amputated. Also, the tendons, nerves, and ligaments that enable normal function and movement of the paw are severed. An analogous procedure applied to humans would be cutting off each finger at the last joint.Declawing, also known as onychectomy, is a major surgical and potentially crippling procedure that robs an animal of its primary means of defense. Declawed animals may be at increased risk of injury or death, if attacked by other animals. They are deprived of their normal, instinctual behavioral impulses to use their claws to climb, exercise, and mark territory with the scent glands in their paws.

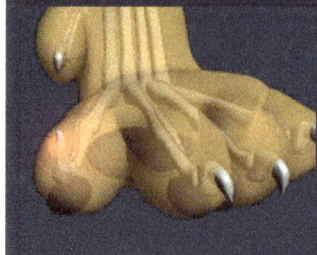

DOES DECLAWING CAUSE PAIN?

Sometimes, the de-knuckling procedure leaves remnants of the nail bed, so claws may grow back again through tender tissue, paw pads and skin, which is very painful.

Declawing is one of the most painful, routinely performed procedures in all of veterinary medicine. Each toe of the cat is amputated at the first joint. Declawing a cat is equivalent in a person to amputating the entire first knuckle of every finger.

Declaw surgery is so predictably painful that it is used by pharmaceutical companies to test the effectiveness of pain medications in clinical trials. Initial recovery after declaw amputation surgery takes a few weeks, but even after the surgical wounds have healed, there are often other long-term physical complications and negative psychological effects. Declaw surgery exposes cats to the risks of general anesthesia and complications of the surgical procedure, which include bleeding, infection, lameness, nerve damage, gangrene, extensive tissue damage and death.

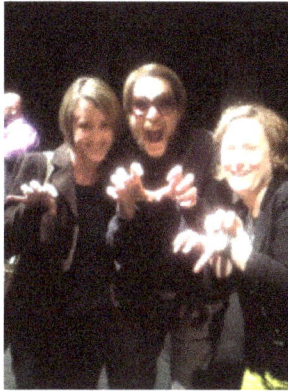

A cat's natural instinct to scratch serves both physical and psychological needs. Their claws are their primary, instinctive tools for defending themselves and capturing prey. They scratch to keep their nails in condition and to mark territory. Before domestication, cats satisfied these needs by clawing tree trunks. House cats can be trained to satisfy their desire to claw without damaging valuable property. Most cats can be trained to use a scratching post. Other options include the use of nail trimmers, sticky strips applied to furniture, climbing trees and scratching mats.

Cats stretch their bodies and tone their muscles by digging their claws into something and pulling back against their own clawhold. Declawed cats are deprived of the means to defend themselves or flee from danger. Declawed cats have been injured or killed by other animals when they could not climb out of harm's way or had impaired ability to protect themselves.

By far, the most common reason given by cat owners who are considering having their pet declawed is to protect furniture or other property. Some may believe that declawing will prevent the cat from injuring them. Some veterinarians will recommend the procedure to their clients. Some people will not ever notice that their cats are having trouble after being declawed. Unfortunately, as many people discover too late, declawing may cause far worse problems than it solves. There are many better ways to treat behavior problems other than radical and irreversible surgery.

Veterinary Surgery

Veterinary surgery is surgery performed on animals by veterinarians, whereby the procedures fall into three broad categories: orthopaedics (bones, joints, muscles), soft tissue surgery (skin, body cavities, cardiovascular system, GI/urogenital/respiratory tracts), and neurosurgery. Advanced surgical procedures such as joint replacement (total hip, knee and elbow replacement), fracture repair, stabilization of cranial cruciate ligament deficiency, oncologic (cancer) surgery, herniated disc treatment, complicated gastrointestinal or urogenital procedures, kidney transplant, skin grafts, complicated wound management, minimally invasive procedures (arthroscopy, laparoscopy, thoracoscopy) are performed by veterinary surgeons (as registered in their jurisdiction). Most general practice veterinarians perform routine surgery [neuters (spay and castration), minor mass excisions, etc.], some also perform additional procedures.

The goal of veterinary surgery may be quite different in pets and in farm animals. In the former, the situation is more close to that with human beings, where the benefit to the patient is the important factor. In the latter, the economic benefit is more important.

Specialization in Surgery

In the United States, Canada and Europe, veterinary surgery is one of 22 veterinary specialties recognized by the American Veterinary Medical Association respectively the European Board of Veterinary Specialisation. Those wishing to become board certified must undergo a one-year clinical internship program followed by three years of intensive training in a residency program under direct supervision of Board Certified Veterinary Surgeons, including performance of a large number of surgical procedures in such categories as abdominal surgery, surgical treatment of angular limb deformities, arthroscopic surgery, surgery of the foot, fracture fixation, ophthalmic surgery, urogenital surgery, and upper respiratory surgery, etc. Once the minimum requirements of training are met residents are required to pass a rigorous certification examination before being admitted as members (Diplomates) of the American College of Veterinary Surgeons or European College of Veterinary Surgeons.

Veterinary Anesthesia

Anesthesia in animals has many similarities to human anesthesia, but some differences as well. Local anesthesia is primarily used for wound closure and removal of small tumors. Lidocaine, mepivacaine, and bupivacaine are the most commonly used local anesthetics used in veterinary medicine. Sedation without general anesthesia is used for more involved procedures. Sedatives commonly used include acepromazine, hydromorphine, midazolam, diazepam, xylazine, and medetomidine. α2 agonists like xylazine and medetomidine are especially useful because they can be reversed, xylazine by yohimbine and medetomidine by atipamezole. Xylazine is approved for use in dogs, cats, horses, deer, and elk in the United States, while medetomidine is only approved for dogs. Most surgeries in ruminants can be performed with regional anesthesia.

General anesthesia is commonly used in animals for major surgery. Animals are often premedicated intravenously or intramuscularly with a sedative, analgesic, and anticholinergic agent (dogs frequently receive buprenorphine, acepromazine, and glycopyrrolate). The next step is induction, usually with an intravenous drug. Dogs and cats commonly receive thiopental (no longer allowed in the UK), ketamine with diazepam, tiletamine with zolazepam (usually just in cats), and/or propofol. Alfaxalone is a steroid anaesthetic used in many practices in the UK to induce anaesthesia in cats and sometimes dogs. It is similar in physiological effect but different in composition to the now withdrawn Saffan. Horses commonly receive thiopental and guaifenesin. Following induction, the animal is intubated with an endotracheal tube and maintained on a gas anesthetic. The most common gas anesthetics in use in veterinary medicine are isoflurane, enflurane, and halothane, although desflurane and sevoflurane are becoming more popular due to rapid induction and recovery.

Common Veterinary Surgeries

Elective Procedures

Elective procedures are those performed on a non-emergency basis, and which do not involve immediately life-threatening conditions. These are in contrast to emergency procedures.

Sterilization Surgery

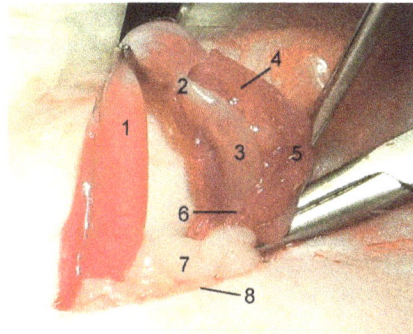

A cat spay

One of the most common elective surgical procedures in animals are those that render animals incapable of reproducing. Neutering in animals describes spaying or castration. To spay (medical term: ovariectomy or ovario-hysterectomy) is to completely remove the ovaries and often the uterus of a female animal. In a dog, this is accomplished through a ventral midline incision into the abdomen. In a cat, this is accomplished either by a ventral midline abdominal incision, or by a flank incision (more common in the UK). With an ovariectomy ligatures are placed on the blood vessels above and below the ovary and the organ is removed. With an ovariohysterectomy, the ligaments of the uterus and ovaries are broken down and the blood vessels are ligated and both organs are removed. The body wall, subcutis, and skin are sutured. To castrate (medical term: orchiectomy) is to remove the testicles of a male animal. Different techniques are used depending on the type of animal, including ligation of the spermatic cord with suture material, placing a rubber band around the cord to restrict blood flow to the testes, or crushing the cord with a specialized instrument like the Burdizzo.

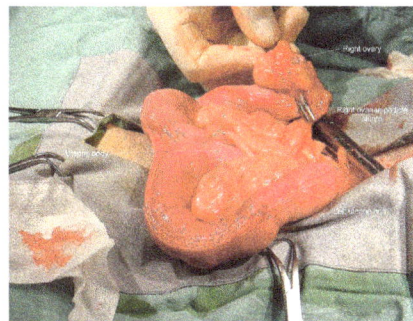

Pyometra surgery

Neutering is usually performed to prevent breeding, prevent unwanted behavior, or decrease risk of future medical problems. Neutering is also performed as an emergency procedure to treat certain reproductive diseases, like pyometra and testicular torsion, and it is used to treat ovarian, uterine, and testicular cancer. It is also recommended in cases of cryptorchidism to prevent torsion and malignant transformation of the testicles.

Laser surgery offers a number of benefits, including reduced risk of infection, less post-operative pain and swelling, reduced bleeding and improved visibility of the surgical field. Better hemostasis and visibility can in some cases minimize the need for anesthesia and/or reduce overall surgical time.

Controversial Elective Animal Procedures

Other common elective surgical procedures in the United States are declawing in cats (onychectomy), ear-cropping in dogs, tail docking in dogs, horses, and dairy cattle, and Livestock dehorning in cattle, sheep, and goats. These procedures have been controversial and recently debated among breeders, veterinary organizations, and animal welfare scientists. The controversy is different for each procedure, but issues arise based on reasons to perform the procedure, differing opinions on techniques and methods, perceived long-term benefits in individual animals, and the development of alternatives. Declawing, for example, consists of removal of the distal phalanges using either a scalpel, scissors or laser. It is typically performed to prevent property damage in house cats, but may also be performed in purebred dogs to meet certain show requirements. Some procedures are illegal in some countries (in the UK, declawing is illegal and tail docking is only allowed in working dogs) and face ethical challenges in others.

Dental Surgery

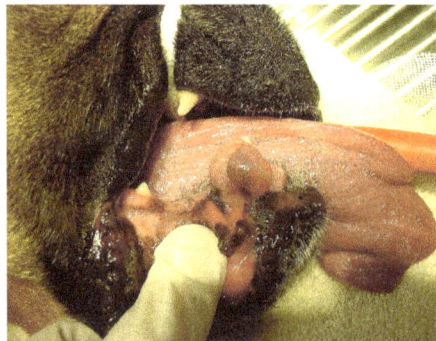
Anesthetised dog with an epulis

Common dental surgical procedures:

- Horses - Floating (grinding down) of uneven teeth edges and removal of wolf teeth.

- Dogs - Dental prophylaxis is commonly performed to remove tartar and treat periodontal disease. This procedure is usually performed under anesthesia. Other common procedures include extraction of abscessed or broken teeth, extraction of deciduous teeth, root canals, and removal of gingival hyperplasia and epulides.

- Cats - Dental prophylaxis as described above for the dog and treatment and extraction of teeth with feline odontoclastic resorptive lesions (FORLs).

Surgical Oncology

In older dogs and cats tumors are a common occurrence, and may involve any or multiple body systems: skin, musculoskeletal, gastrointestinal tract, urogentital tract, reproductive tract, cardiovascular system, spinal cord and peripheral nerves, the spleen and the lining of body cavities. Common skin tumors include lipomas, mast cell tumors, melanomas, squamous cell carcinomas, basal cell carcinomas, fibrosarcomas, and histiocytomas. Skin tumors are removed through either simple excisions or through excisions needing reconstructive plastic surgery. Common oral tumors include melanomas, fibrosarcomas, squamous cell carcinomas, which are removed with as much surrounding tissue as possible, including parts of the mandible and maxilla. Other types of cancer requiring surgery include osteosarcoma, stomach and intestinal tumors, splenic masses, and urinary bladder tumors.

Ophthalmic Surgery

Common ophthalmic surgeries in animals include:

- Enucleation of the eye to treat glaucoma or eye proptosis
- Cataract surgery
- Entropion surgery
- Ectropion surgery
- Eyelid tumor removal
- Cherry eye surgery
- Exenteration (complete removal) of the orbit, especially for squamous cell carcinoma in the cat and cow.

Orthopedic Surgery

Common orthopedic surgeries in animals include:

- Ruptured anterior cruciate ligament repair
- For hip dysplasia:
  - Femoral head ostectomy
  - Triple pelvic osteotomy
  - Hip replacement
- Leg amputation
- Bone fracture repair
- Arthroscopy

- MPL - medial patellar luxation

- APL - anterior patellar luxation.

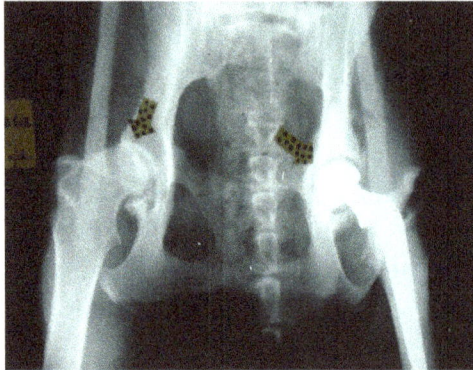
X-ray of a dog with an artificial hip to repair hip dysplasia

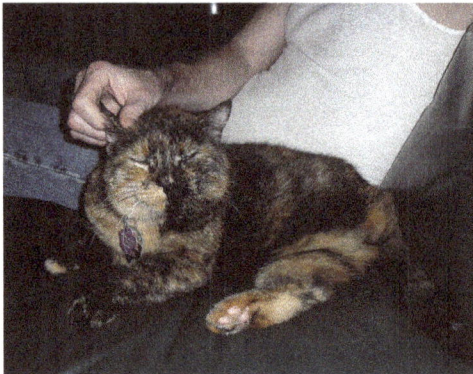
A healthy tortoise-mix cat healed and adapted quickly to her new mobility after a hind leg was amputated

Cardiology Surgery

Common cardiology surgeries in animals include:

- Balloon Valvuloplasty: Procedure used to alleviate pain symptoms from cardiac problems such as pulmonic, mitral, and tricuspid stenosis. The purpose of this procedure is to create a more smooth blood flow throughout the body by reducing harmful symptoms from obstructed heart valves. It is considered a minimally invasive procedure. The procedure involves putting a balloon-like object inside of the animal's heart, the balloon inflates and deflates in order to alleviate pain and increase blood flow. This procedure is not anything major but complications can occur if the animals body rejects the balloon and could form a life-threatening allergic reaction.

- Centesis: Procedure consisting of the removal of fluid from an animal's body in order to manage congestive heart failure. By draining fluid, it helps prevent tumors from growing around the heart. Animals undergo no anesthesia because no little pain occurs during this operation. Catheters and needles of various sizes will be punctured through the animal's body. To remove the actual fluid, vets will use a syringe suction or vacuum. Post-op, swelling might occur around the thoracic cavity or appear bruised but this is normal and is rarely discomforting to the animal.

- • Devive Embolization of Persistent Ductus Arteriosus (PDA): PDA is caused by an un-normal blood flow from right to left inside the heart. This causes patients to develop left-sided congestive heart failure. In order to help fix this, coils are placed inside ducts of the heart. The coils embolize into the pulmonary arteries. ACDO devices are not expensive and the procedure itself is not expensive.

Other Common Procedures

Caesarean Section

Caesarean sections are commonly performed in dogs, cats, horses, sheep, and cattle. Usually it is done as an emergency surgery due to difficulties in the birthing process. Certain dog breeds such as Bulldogs often need to have this surgery because of the size of the puppy's head relative to the width of the bitch's birth canal.

Surgery for Gastric Dilatation Volvulus (Bloat)

Gastric dilatation volvulus (bloat) is a common condition in dogs in which the stomach fills with gas, and can become torsed. This requires immediate surgical intervention to prevent necrosis of the stomach wall and death of the dog. During surgery, the stomach is deflated and put back into its normal position. A gastropexy may be performed, whereby the stomach is attached to the body wall to prevent this condition from recurring. A splenectomy or partial gastrectomy may also be required.

Cystotomy

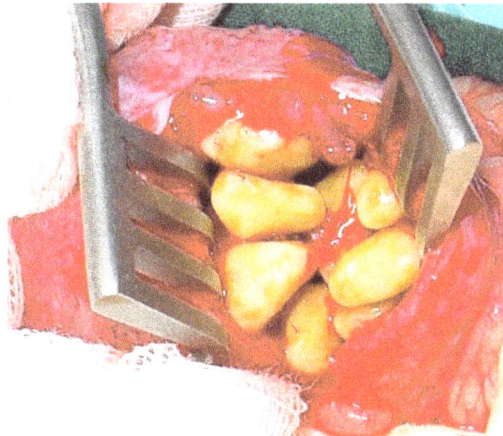

Cystotomy to remove bladder stones

A cystotomy is a surgical opening of the urinary bladder. It is commonly performed in dogs and cats to remove bladder stones or tumors.

Wound Repair

Bite wounds from other animals (and rarely humans) are a common occurrence. Wounds from objects that the animal may step on or run into are also common. Usually these wounds are simple lacerations that can be easily cleaned and sutured, sometimes using a local anesthetic. Bite wounds, however, involve compressive and tensile forces in addition to shearing forces, and can cause separation of the skin from the underlying tissue and avulsion of underlying muscles. Deep puncture wounds are especially prone to infection. Deeper wounds are assessed under anesthesia and explored, lavaged, and debrided. Primary wound closure is used if all remaining tissue is healthy and free of contamination. Small puncture wounds may be left open, bandaged, and allowed to heal without surgery. A third alternative is delayed primary closure, which involves bandaging and reevaluation and surgery in three to five days.

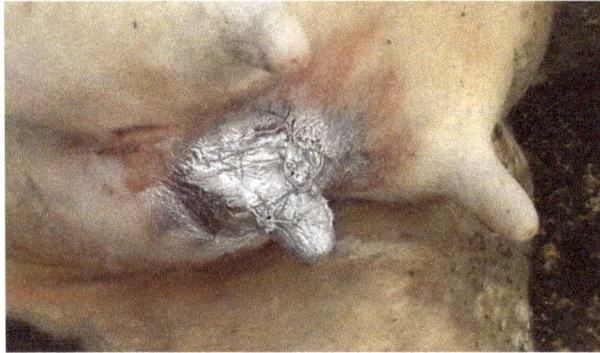
Sutured wound on the teats of a cow

Wounds occurring in the udder and teats of cows are more difficult to repair, due to the difficult access and sensitivity of the organ, and because deep anaesthesia may not be applied to bovines. But some practitioners have acquired a great experience in dealing them.

Foreign Body Removal

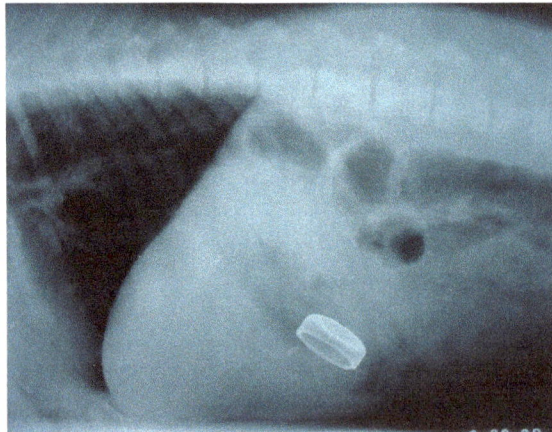
Bottle top swallowed by a dog that had to be removed surgically

A variety of non-edible objects are commonly swallowed by dogs, cats, and cattle. These foreign bodies can cause obstruction of the gastrointestinal tract causing severe vomiting and resulting electrolyte imbalances. The stomach (gastrotomy) or intestine (enterotomy) can be surgically opened to remove the foreign body. Necrotic intestine can be removed (enterectomy) and repaired with intestinal anastomosis. Foreign bodies can also be removed by endoscopy, which although requires general anesthesia does not require surgery and significantly decreases recovery time. However, endoscopic foreign body retrieval is anatomically limited to objects lodged in the esophagus, the stomach or the colon. The condition in cattle is known as hardware disease.

Organ Replacement in Animals

Limb replacement (prosthesis) in animals is a well developed science and becoming more common. Organ replacement is rarer and much more difficult. The first pacemaker surgery on a dog was performed in 1968. About 300 pacemakers are implanted in dogs each year. Successful kidney transplants in cats have been around since the mid-1980's. Canine programs have been less successful due to the problems of immunosuppression. The way donor animals are treated remains a source of concern.

Kidney Transplantation

Kidney transplantation has so far only been performed with any degree of success on cats and dogs, most usually cats as they are particularly prone to kidney diseases. The School of Veterinary Medicine at U.C. Davis initiated the Renal Transplantation Program in 1987. Cats can tolerate transplantation from unrelated cats, but must be supported with immunosuppressive drugs for the rest of their lives. When the transplanted kidney is implanted in the recipient the original kidneys are usually left in place.

There are currently ten centers in the world that offer kidney transplants for cats. Most are in the US. UC Davis have since abandoned their program. Kidney transplantation is a controversial treatment option, with longevity, quality of life, as well as ethical considerations. Many argue that it causes unnecessary suffering to donor animals.

Total Hip Replacement

A good candidate for total hip replacement (THR) must be at least 9–12 months old to be sure he has finished developing and weigh at least 30 pounds (14 kg). The hip implant for dogs is similar to its human counterpart, but it is much smaller. X-rays are used to determine the dimensions of an appropriately sized implant.

The femoral stem is usually made of cobalt chrome or stainless steel, while the cup is made of ultra high molecular weight polyethylene. Polymethyl methacrylate is the cement used with cemented implants, whereas 250-micrometres (diameter) titanium beads usually cover the stem surface of the press-fit implants.

The THR is expected to last 10–15 years, which usually surpasses the remaining lifetime of the dog. In less than 5% of cases, the THR will malfunction through loosening of the acetabular cup or femoral fracture. These failures require correction with revision surgery.

Pacemaker Implants

The first pacemaker surgery on a dog was performed in 1968. About 300 pacemakers are implanted in dogs each year, even though about 4000 dogs are in need of one. There are no pacemakers made specifically for use in dogs, but human pacemaker users are often outlasted by their pacemakers, leaving behind a functioning pacemaker with less battery power left than a new pacemaker which could be implanted into a dog. One difficulty in implanting used pacemakers is the removal from the deceased human - the pacemaker leads often experience accumulation of surrounding heart muscle tissue and become difficult to remove after death. If the leads are cut in order to remove the pacemaker donation is not possible. If a pacemaker has not been used by a human but has reached its expiry date it will not be suitable for use in a human but could still be used in a dog.

Blood Transfusion

For a blood transfusion to take place, the donor and recipient must be of compatible blood types. Dogs have eleven blood types but are born without antibodies in their blood. For this reason, first time transfusions will not have a reaction, but further transfusions will cause severe reactions if the dog has a mismatch in the DEA1.1 blood type. Because the immune systems of dogs are so fierce, cross-match tests must be performed upon each dog blood transfusion. Only about one in every 15 dogs is negative for all antigens and thus, a universal donor. Cats have A, B, and AB blood types with specific factors, but there is no universal donor type Recipient and donor blood must be properly cross-matched. Red cells from the donor are mixed with the serum of the recipient in major cross-matching. In a minor cross-match, the recipient's red cells are compared with the donor's serum. Blood donors must meet specific requirements in order to qualify to donate. They must weigh at least 50 lb for dogs and 10 lb for cats, have high enough blood component values, and have no infectious diseases. One donation could be used by up to two animals.

Policy regarding how donor animals are treated varies. In April, 2014, a veterinarian office in Fort Worth Texas, was accused of keeping dogs that had been presumed to have been euthanized, and using the animals for blood withdrawal.

Heart Valves

Open-heart surgery for dogs requires a six- to eight-person team to carefully monitor the patient before and during the invasive surgery. The entire surgery lasts five hours, during which time the dog is connected to a blood oxygenator and the heart is bypassed. The defective heart valve is removed and the replacement valve, typically from bovine pericardium, is precisely sewn into place. The dog's heart is then restarted and monitored for at least two hours after the surgery is completed. Due to the expense, this is not a common procedure.

Prosthetic Limbs

While small dogs and cats can survive comfortably with three legs, larger dogs, horses, and farm animals require the limb to support their weight. Surgery has also been done on birds that are used for breeding purposes. Each prosthetic limb is custom-made to fit the individual needs of the specific animal.

Orthopedic Implants

UC Davis' equine orthopedic surgery program has developed an implant that has been successful in human surgery for a long time. The intermedullary interlocking nail is used to treat horses with long leg bone fractures. The nails are positioned within the medullary cavity and can be secured to the proximal and distal fracture segments using transcortical screws which penetrate both cortices of the bone, as well as pass through holes in the nail. The nail is placed centrally in the axis of the bone to give full support unlike bone plates that only give exterior support. In an attempt to aid horses with bowed tendons, research has been done using carbon fiber implants that consist of about 40,000 fibers in total each of which is 8 micrometres in diameter. These fibers induce tissue growth and result in a structure of carbon and tissue about 8 mm in diameter.

Devocalization

Devocalization (also known as ventriculocordectomy or vocal cordectomy and when performed on dogs is commonly known as debarking or bark softening) is a surgical procedure performed on dogs and cats, where tissue is removed from the animal's vocal cords to permanently reduce the volume of its vocalizations.

Indications and Contraindications

Devocalization is usually performed at the request of an animal owner (where the procedure is legally permitted). The procedure may be forcefully requested as a result of a court order. Owners or breeders generally request the procedure because of excessive animal vocalizations, complaining neighbors, or as an alternative to euthanasia due to a court order.

Contraindications include negative reaction to anesthesia, infection, bleeding, and pain. There is also the possibility of the removed tissue growing back, or of scar tissue blocking the throat, both requiring further surgeries, though with the incisional technique, the risk of fibrosis is virtually eliminated.

Effectiveness

Canine

The devocalization procedure does not take away a dog's ability to bark. Dogs will normally bark just as much as before the procedure. After the procedure the sound will be softer, typically about half as loud as before, or less, and it is not as sharp or piercing. So while the procedure does not stop barking or silence the animal completely, it is effective in reducing the sound level and sharpness of the dog's bark.

Most devocalized dogs have a subdued "husky" bark, audible up to 20 metres.

Surgical Procedure

The procedure may be performed via the animal's mouth, with a portion of the vocal folds removed using a biopsy punch, cautery tool, scissor, or laser. The procedure may also be performed via an incision in the throat and through the larynx, which is a more invasive technique. All devocalization procedures require general anesthesia.

Reasons for Excessive Vocalization

Chronic, excessive vocalization may be due to improper socialization or training, stress, boredom, fear, or frustration. Up to 35% of dog owners report problems with barking, which can cause disputes and legal problems. The behavior is more common among some breeds of dog, such as the Shetland Sheepdog, which are known as loud barkers, due to the nature of the environment in which the breed was developed.

Less Invasive Interventions

Vocalizations are a natural behavior of animals which they use widely in intra-specific and inter-specific communication. As such, devocalization should generally be considered only as a last resort. Prior to this surgical intervention, there are other, less invasive interventions which can be considered to overcome excessive vocalizations.

Training

Training can be one of the most effective techniques to help combat excessive barking in dogs. Acquiring the help of a professional dog trainer can often help reduce an animal's barking.

Corrective Collars

The use of automatic and manual corrective collars can be useful as a training aid when used correctly; however, the use of corrective collars, particularly shock collars, is controversial and banned in some countries. Types of corrective collars include vibration, citronella spray, ultrasonic and electrostatic/shock collar.

Accommodation

Because dogs often bark excessively due to stress, boredom, or frustration, changing aspects of an animal's environment to make them more content is a suitable way to quiet them down, rather than forcibly silencing a distressed animal. Spending more time with an animal, such as playing, walking, and other bonding activities, will keep them occupied and make them feel more at ease. If the animal is stressed, it is best to remove the object that is causing them discomfort.

Cropping

Cropping is the removal of part or all of the pinnae or auricles, the external visible flap of the ear and earhole, of an animal; it sometimes involves taping to make the ears pointy. Most commonly performed on dogs, it is an ancient practice that was once done for perceived health, practical or cosmetic reasons. In modern times, it is banned in many nations, but is still legal in a limited number of countries. Where permitted, it is seen only in certain breeds of dog such as the Pit bull, Miniature Pinscher, German Pinscher, Doberman Pinscher, Schnauzer, Great Dane, Boxer, Bouvier des Flandres, Neapolitan Mastiff, Cane Corso, Perro de Presa Canario, Dogo Argentino, Caucasian Shepherd Dog, Central Asian Shepherd Dog and Beauceron.

The veterinary procedure is known as cosmetic otoplasty. Current veterinary science provides no medical or physical advantage to the animal from the procedure, leading to concerns over animal cruelty related to performing unnecessary surgery on the animals. In addition to the bans in place in countries around the world, it is described in some veterinary texts as "no longer considered ethical."

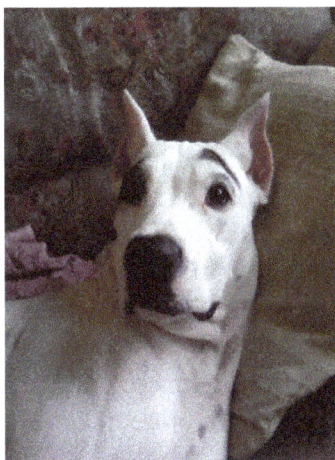

A Guatemalan Dogo with cropped ears

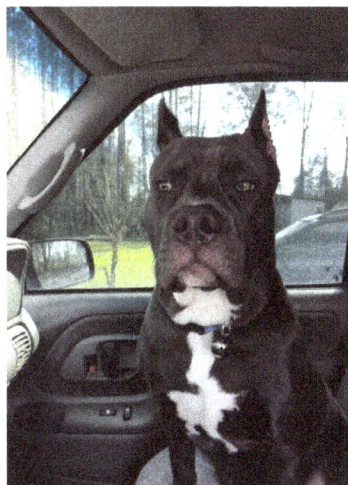

Pit bull with cropped ears

Cropping of large portions of the pinnae of other animals is rare, although the clipping of identifying shapes in the pinnae of livestock, called earmarks, was common prior to the introduction of compulsory ear tags. Removal of portions of the ear of laboratory mice for identification, i.e. ear-notching, is still used. The practice of cropping for cosmetic purposes is rare in non-canines, although some selectively bred animals have naturally small ears which can be mistaken for cropping.

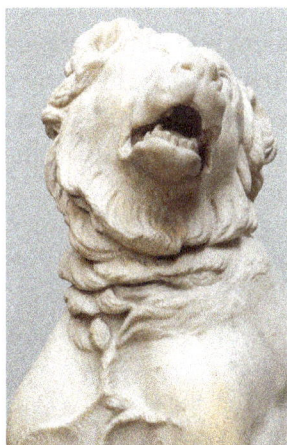

The Duncombe Dog, a 2nd-century AD Roman copy of a Hellenistic bronze, probably of the 2nd century BC and from Epirus, showing cropped ears

Ear cropping has been performed on dogs since ancient times.

Traditional Cropping

Historically, cropping was performed on working dogs in order to decrease the risk of health complications, such as ear infections or hematomas. Crops were also performed on dogs that might need to fight, either while hunting animals that might fight back or while defending livestock herds from predators, or because they were used for pit-fighting sports such as dogfighting or bear-baiting. The ears were an easy target for an opposing animal to grab or tear.

Cropping the ears of livestock guardian dogs was, and may still be, traditional in some pastoral cultures. The ears of working flock-defense dogs such as the Caucasian Shepherd Dog (Kavka-zskaïa Ovtcharka) and the Pastore Maremmano-Abruzzese were traditionally cropped to reduce the possibility of wolves or aggressor dogs getting a hold on them. According to one description, cropping was carried out when puppies were weaned, at about six weeks. It was performed by an older or expert shepherd, using the ordinary blade shears used for shearing, well sharpened. The ears were cut either to a point like those of a fox, or rounded like those of a bear. The removed auricles were given to the puppy to eat, in the belief that it would make him more "sour"; the ears were first grilled. An alternative method was to remove the ears from newborn puppies by twisting them off; however, this left almost no external ear on the dog. More than three hundred years ago, both ear-cropping and the use of spiked collars,because wolves could have a hard time choking the dog out, were described as a defense against wolves by Jean de la Fontaine in Fable 9 of Book X of the *Fables*, published in 1678.

Dogs may have their ears cropped, legally or not, for participation in dogfights, themselves illegal in many jurisdictions.

Health Benefits

Historically, ear cropping has been advocated as a health benefit for certain breeds with long, hanging ears. It used to be believed, and was wrongly so, that dogs with standing ears may suffer from fewer ear infections than dogs with hanging ears, but this is dated and not a sensible reason for an animal to undertake this surgery. It has also been hypothesized that standing ears are less prone to damage and subsequent medical complications, especially in working dogs. Some claim that cropped ears enhance Boxers' hearing. Long, hanging ears can not function the same way as erect ears which can swivel toward a sound source. The erect shape directs sound waves into the ear canal and additionally amplifies the sound slightly. Long, hanging pinnae also impose a physical barrier to sound waves entering the ear canal.

Cosmetic Cropping

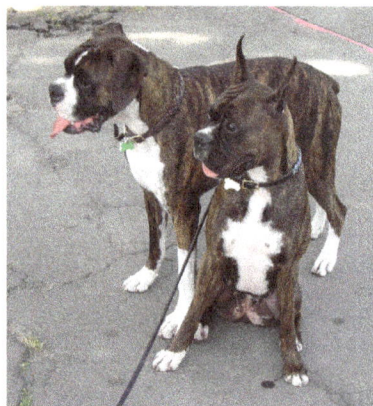

Boxers with natural and cropped ears and docked tails

In the last 100 years or so, ear cropping has been performed more often for cosmetic purposes. In nations and states where it remains legal, it is usually practiced because it is required as part of a breed standard for exhibition at dog shows.

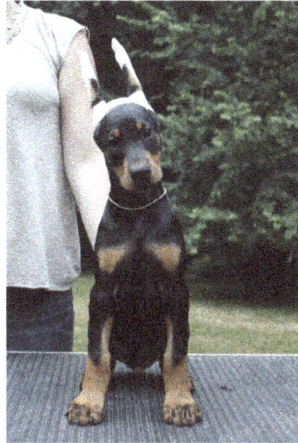

A Doberman Pinscher puppy with its ears taped to train them into
the desired shape and carriage after cropping

The veterinary procedure is known as "cosmetic otoplasty". It is usually performed on puppies at 7 to 12 weeks of age. After 16 weeks, the procedure is more painful and the animal has greater pain memory. Up to 2/3 of the ear flap may be removed in a cropping operation, and the wound edges are closed with stitches. The ears are then bandaged and taped until they heal into the proper shape. The procedure is recommended to be undertaken under general anaesthesia; opponents' primary concerns revolve around post-operative pain.

American veterinary schools do not generally teach cropping and docking, and thus veterinarians who perform the practice have to learn on the job. There are also problems with amateurs performing ear-cropping, particularly at puppy mills.

In the USA, although tail-docking, dewclaw removal, and neutering procedures remain common, ear-cropping is declining, save within the dog show industry. However, many show ring competitors state they would discontinue the practice altogether if they could still "win in the ring."

Animal Welfare and Law

The practice is illegal across most of Europe, including all countries that have ratified the European Convention for the Protection of Pet Animals, and most member countries of the Fédération Cynologique Internationale. It is illegal in parts of Spain and in some Canadian provinces. The situation in Italy is unclear; the ban effective 14 January 2007 may no longer be in force.

Ear-cropping is still widely practiced in the United States and parts of Canada, with approximately 130,000 puppies in the United States thought to have their ears cropped each year. The American and Canadian Kennel Clubs both permit the practice. The American Kennel Club (AKC) position is that ear cropping and tail docking are "acceptable practices integral to defining and preserving breed character and/or enhancing good health." While some individual states have attempted to ban ear-cropping, there is strong opposition from some dog breed organizations, who cite health concerns and tradition.

The American Veterinary Medical Association "opposes ear cropping and tail docking of dogs when done solely for cosmetic purposes" and "encourages the elimination of ear cropping and tail docking from breed standards". Specifically, the AVMA "has recommended to the American Kennel Club and appropriate breed associations that action be taken to delete mention of cropped or trimmed ears from breed standards for dogs and to prohibit the showing of dogs with cropped or trimmed ears if such animals were born after some reasonable date". Some national chains of veterinary hospitals have voluntarily ceased to perform cosmetic surgeries on dogs. The American Humane Association opposes ear-cropping "unless it is medically necessary, as determined by a licensed veterinarian".

While it has been suggested the cropping may interfere with a dog's ability to communicate using ear signals, some also argue that cropping increases a dog's ability to communicate with ear signals. There has been no scientific comparative study of ear communication in cropped and uncropped dogs.

Naturally Small Ears

Some animals, such as the Lamancha goat, have ears which are naturally small as the result of selective breeding, and some people mistakenly believe their ears to be cropped.

In other animals, small ears may result from a genetic mutation or the emergence of a genetically recessive trait, such as in Highland cattle, where the appearance of small ears, appearing to have their pinnae cropped, is viewed as a defect.

Docking

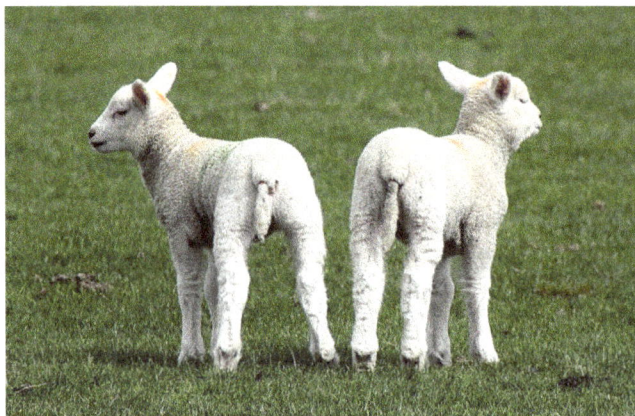

Two lambs having their tails docked by the use of rubber rings for elastration. The tight rubber rings block blood flow to the lower portion of the tail, which will atrophy and fall off

Docking is the intentional removal of part of an animal's tail or, sometimes, ears. The term cropping is more commonly used in reference to the cropping of ears, while *docking* more commonly—but not exclusively—refers to the tail. The term tailing is also commonly used. The term arises because the living flesh of the tail, from which the animal's tail hairs grow, commonly is known as the dock.

Dogs

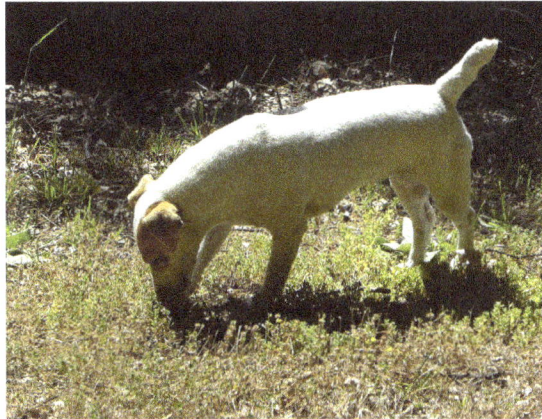

Dog with partially docked tail sniffing for truffles

As with other domesticated animals there is a long history of docking the tails of dogs. It is understood to date at least to the Roman Empire. The most popular reason for docking dog breeds is to prevent injury to working dogs. In hunting dogs, the tail is docked to prevent it from getting cut up as the dog wags its tail in the brush. This is contested by a wide range of groups and is sometimes considered a form of animal cruelty. This has led to the practice being outlawed and made illegal throughout many countries, in some of which dogs are no longer bred for work, or used as working animals.

For example, in United Kingdom tail docking was originally undertaken largely by dog breeders. However, in 1991, the UK government amended the Veterinary Surgeons Act, prohibiting the docking of dogs' tails by lay persons from 1 July 1993. Only veterinary surgeons were, by law, allowed to dock. However, following the passage of the law, the Council of the Royal College of Veterinary Surgeons in November 1992, ruled docking to be unethical, "unless for therapeutic or acceptable prophylactic reasons". The requirement in which the Royal College considers prophylactic docking to be acceptable are so strict as to make the routine docking of puppies by veterinary surgeons extremely difficult. Vets who continue to dock risk disciplinary action, and can be removed from the professional register. Those found guilty of unlawful docking would face a fine of up to £20,000, up to 51 weeks imprisonment or both. They can only dock the tail of "working" dogs (in some specific cases) - e.g. hunting dogs that work in areas thick in brambles and heavy vegetation where the dog's tail can get caught and cause injury to the dog. Docking was banned in England and Wales by the Animal Welfare Act 2006 and in Scotland by the Animal Health and Welfare (Scotland) Act 2006.

In 1987 the European Convention for the Protection of Pet Animals, established by Council of Europe, prohibited docking for non-medical reasons, though signatory countries are free to opt out of this provision, and almost half of them have done so. Norway completely banned the practice in 1987. Other countries where docking is banned include Australia and the United Kingdom.

Horses

Originally, most docking was done for practical purposes. For example, a draft horse used for hauling large loads might have had its tail docked to prevent it from becoming entangled in tow ropes, farm machinery, or harness; without docking, it could be dangerous to the horse, painful if the tail were tangled, and inconvenient to the owner to tie up the horse's tail for every use.

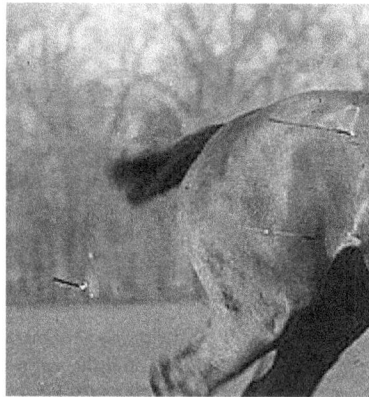

Docked and banged tail on a polo pony

In modern use, the term usually does not refer to tail amputation as it does with some dog breeds. However, historically, docking was performed on some horses, often as foals. The practice has been banned in some nations, but is still seen on some show and working draft horses in some places, and is practiced at some PMU operations.

In modern times, the term "docked" or "docking" in reference to the tail of a horse generally refers to the practice of cutting the hair of the tail skirt very short, just past the end of the natural dock of the tail. In particular, the tail is often cut short to keep it from being tangled in a harness.

Cattle

Tail docking of dairy cows is prevalent in some regions. Some anecdotal reports have suggested that such docking may reduce SCC (somatic cell counts in milk) and occurrence of mastitis. However, a study examining such issues found no significant effect of docking on SCC or mastitis frequency or on four measures of cow cleanliness. Although it has been suggested that leptospirosis among dairy farm workers might be reduced by docking cows' tails, a study found that milkers' leptospiral titers were not related to tail docking. The American Veterinary Medical Association opposes "routine tail docking of cattle." Similarly, the Canadian Veterinary Medical Association opposes docking tails of dairy cattle.

Cattle on large Australian cattle stations often have the tail brush (not the dock) cut shorter (banged) before their release; this "bang-tail muster" indicates those having been counted, treated, their current pregnancy status determined, etc.

Tail docking in the dairy industry is prohibited in Denmark, Germany, Scotland, Sweden, the United Kingdom, and some Australian states, as well as California, Ohio, and Rhode Island. Several large organizations within the dairy industry are against tail docking because of the lack of scientific evidence supporting claims benefiting the practice. Scientific studies have demonstrated that there are numerous animal welfare issues with this practice (such as distress, pain, increased activity in pain receptors in the tail stump, abnormal growths of nerve fibers, sensitivity to heat and cold, and clostridial diseases). Fortunately, there is an effective and humane alternative to tail docking, which is switch trimming.

Pigs

In the case of domestic pigs, where commercially raised animals are kept in close quarters, tail docking is performed to prevent injury or to prevent animals from chewing or biting each other's tails.

Urethrostomy

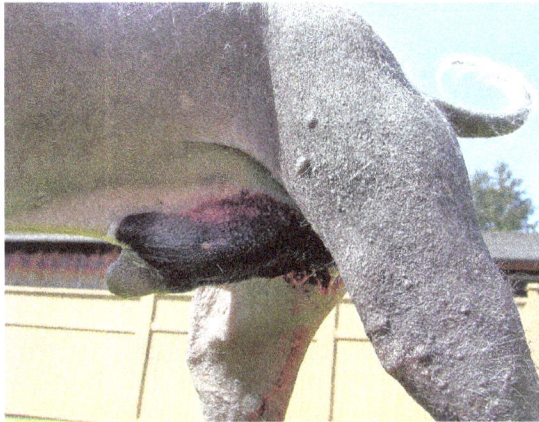
Recently completed scrotal urethrostomy on a dog

Urethrostomy is a surgical procedure that creates a permanent opening in the urethra, commonly to remove obstructions to urine flow. The procedure is most often performed in male cats, where the opening is made in the perineum.

For many years perineal urethrostomy has been used in cattle, sheep and goats, especially young males that have been castrated at a young age, for obstruction by uroliths. However, the anatomy of the male cat is quite different and the urethra is very small in diameter.

Pre-surgical Considerations

Since animals are potentially suffering from severe metabolic derangements at the time of initial presentation, animals need to be stabilized prior to surgery. Common physiologic derangements noted on bloodwork are elevated kidneys values (azotemia) and elevated potassium levels (hyperkalemia). The presence of profound sedation, low body temperature, and/or a slow heart rate (bradycardia) are usually associated with more severe blood derangements.

Ideally, the urethral obstruction is removed or temporarily bypassed with urethral flushing (urohydropulsion) and the placement of an in-dwelling urinary catheter prior to surgery. This catheter allows urine to be removed from the body, and, along with fluid therapy, help normalize blood derangements to resolve prior to anesthesia. There are many types of catheters commonly used, including common red rubber catheters, stiff Tomcat catheters, soft and flexible Cook catheters or semi-rigid "Slippery Sam" catheters.

Sedation is usually required for urohydropulsion and the placement of a urinary catheter due to the associated pain with the procedure. A combination of injectable ketamine and diazepam is a safer option for sedation considering its reduced cardiopulmary depression effects compared to other anesthetics. A combination of etomidate and diazepam would be an even safer anesthetic consideration, but etomidate is not commonly carried by general veterinary practitioners due to its cost.

Fluid therapy is equally essential for correcting derangements. Commonly, a fluid low in potassium, such as 0.9% NaCl, is selected. If 0.9% NaCl is not available, any other crystalloid fluid is realistic even if it contains some level of potassium. Insulin is sometimes used intravenously to temporarily reduce high potassium levels. Calcium gluconate can also be used to protect the myocardium (heart muscle) from the negative effects of hyperkalemia.

Rarely, an urethral obstruction cannot not be removed on initial presentation and emergency surgery must be performed immediately to return urethral patency and save the animal's life. These animals are at a much higher risk under anesthesia.

Surgical Technique

The cat can be placed in either dorsal or ventral recumbency. An elliptical incision is made around the base of the cat's penis and scrotum. If the cat has not been neutered previously, it must be neutered before the perineal urethrostomy can be performed. A combination of sharp and blunt dissection is started ventrally (the underside of the penis) to expose the penis' muscular and soft tissue attachments to the pelvis. After removing these soft tissue attachments to the pelvis, dissection is continued dorsally (on top of the penis) to remove the dorsal retractor penile muscle and other soft tissue covering the site of the required urethral incision.

All of these dissection steps are necessary to free the penis from the pelvis, allowing the veterinarian to move the significantly wider pelvic urethra caudally (or rearward) so it can be attached to the skin.

After the penile body is freed, a dorsal incision is started at the tip of the penis using either a small scalpel blade or fine ophthalmic scissors. This incision is extended to a level at or above the bulbourethral glands. At this level, the urethra is considered wide enough to create an adequate stoma, or urethral opening. The urethra is sutured to the skin for approximately 2 cm using a fine suture on a taper needle. The remainder of the penis is amputated and any remaining skin defect is closed.

As the surgery site heals, the urethral mucosa and skin will heal together creating a permanent stoma. This stoma (opening) is much larger than the original penile urethra making it unlikely for the animal to obstruct in the future.

A urinary catheter may be placed following surgery for the initial 12–24 hours of recovery. This catheter should not be left in longer than this though, as it will increase the likelihood of stricture formation at the surgery site. Animals should wear an e-collar until sutures are removed in 10–14 days.

Post-operative Complications

Initial post-operative complications include wound infection and excessive pain or bleeding. These can be controlled commonly with appropriate prescription medications or ice packs if the animal will tolerate them. A more concerning, though not common, complication is stricture, or narrowing, of the surgery site. The formation of a stricture will require additional procedures to either try and salvage the initial surgery site or create a new urethral opening (or stoma) under the floor of the pelvis (subpelvic urethrostomy) or immediately in front of the pubic bone (pre-pubic urethrostomy).

The most common long term complication associated with this surgery is an increased incidence of urinary tract infections.

Nose Ring

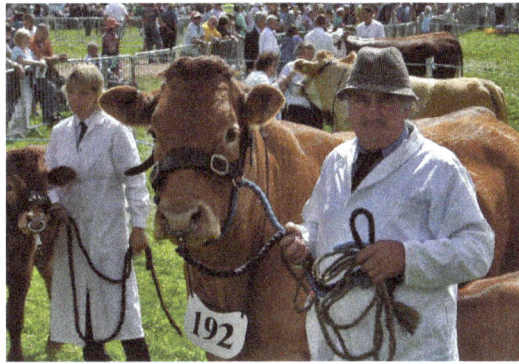

Show halters and bulldog nose rings on cattle at an agricultural show in the United Kingdom

A nose ring is a ring made of metal designed to be installed through the nasal septum of pigs (to prevent them from rooting) as well as domestic cattle, usually bulls. In pigs, nose rings are alternatively pierced through the rim of the nose. Nose rings are often required for bulls when exhibited at agricultural shows. There is a clip-on ring design used for controlling and directing cattle for handling. Nose rings are used to encourage the weaning of young calves by discouraging them from suckling.

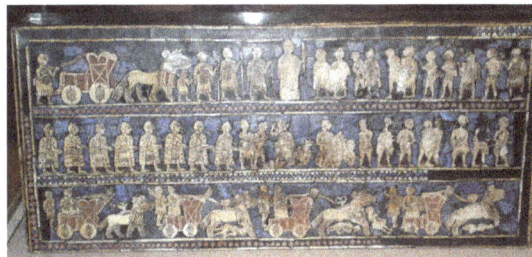

The Standard of Ur

Historically, the use of nose rings for controlling animals dates to the dawn of recorded human civilization. They were used in ancient Sumer and are seen on the Standard of Ur, where they were used on both bovines and equines.

Use

The nose ring assists the handler to control a dangerous animal with minimal risk of injury or disruption by exerting stress on one of the most sensitive parts of the animal, the nose. Bulls, especially, are powerful and sometimes unpredictable animals which, if uncontrolled, can kill or severely injure a human handler.

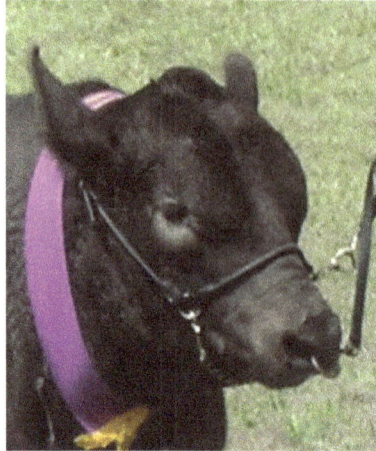

A nose ring is used to maintain control of this bull being exhibited at a livestock show

Control of the bull may be done by holding the ring by hand, looping a piece of rope through it, clipping on a bull staff. A rope or chain from the ring may be attached to a bull's horns or to a head-collar for additional control.

With an aggressive bull, a short length of chain or rope may be left hanging loose from the ring, so when he ducks in a threatening manner, the bull will step on the chain and be deterred from attacking. This lead may also facilitate capture and control of a frisky bull.

Construction and Insertion

Bull rings are usually about 3 to 5 inches (8 to 13 cm) in diameter, depending on the size of the bull. Bull rings are commonly made from aluminium, stainless steel or copper, in the form of a pair of hinged semicircles, held closed by a small brass bolt whose head is broken off during installation. If a ring needs to be removed (for example, if the bull has grown out of it), it is cut or unscrewed.

The ring is normally placed on the bull between 9 and 12 months of age. It is usually done by a veterinarian, who pierces the septum with a scalpel or punch. Self-piercing rings (with sharp ends designed to be pressed through the septum and then pulled together with a screw) have been available for many years; these are also usually installed by a veterinarian rather than the owner.

Other Designs

Calf-weaning Ring

Calf-weaning nose rings or nosebands provide an alternative to separating calves from their mothers during the weaning period. They have plastic spikes which are uncomfortable for the mother, causing her to reject the calf's efforts at suckling. Weaning nose rings are also available for sheep and goats. These nose rings (usually made of plastic) clip onto the nose without piercing it, and are reusable.

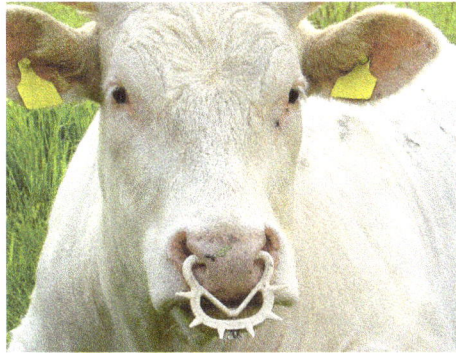

A spiked ring which prevents suckling

Bulldogs

Self-locking or spring-closing show-lead nose rings, also called "bulldogs" or nose grips, are removable rings that do not require the nose to be pierced. They are often used on steers and cows, along with a halter, at agricultural shows, or when handling cattle for examination, marking or treatment. They stay shut until released, and usually have a loop for the attachment of a cord or lead rope. They give similar control to a bull ring without the need for permanent attachment.

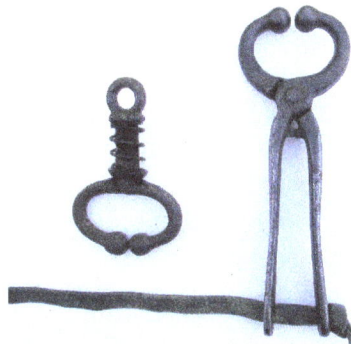

Show-lead nose ring (bulldogs), and bull tongs or bull-holders on the right

Bull Tongs

Bull-holders, also known as bull-tongs, have a pliers action and are used for short periods on grown cattle when they are being mouthed or drenched. A chain, rope or strap keeps the grips closed and may be passed over a bar at the front of a head bail to elevate the head. The thumb and forefinger may also used in this way on smaller animals.

Pig Nose Rings

Rooting is the act of a pig nudging into something with its snout, such as into the dirt to unearth plants to eat. In some circumstances, owners of pigs may find this undesirable. Nose rings make rooting painful for the animal, although a ringed pig may still able to forage freely through leaf litter and surface vegetation. Pig nose-ringing may sometimes be required by local regulations, as when farm pigs are released into public woods to pannage.

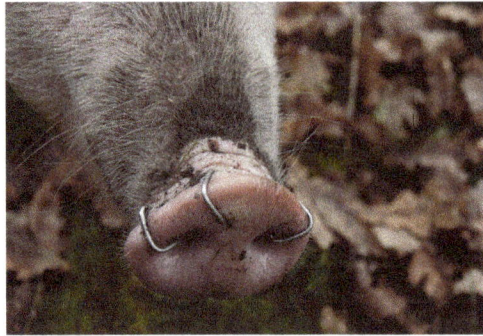
Nose rings on a young pig foraging on the new forest

Nose rings specifically designed for pigs usually consist of open copper or steel wire rings with sharp ends, about one inch (about 2.5 cm) in diameter. These are typically clipped to the rim of the nose instead of through the septum, as this is far more painful to the pig and is considered "thus more effective for deterring the pig from rooting than piercing through the septum is". As they may sometimes become dislodged, an adult pig may be given three to four rings.

Bull Handling in the Show Ring

For safety reasons, many show societies require bulls over 12 months to be led with a nose ring. A bull may be led by a rope tied through the ring, although a halter (headcollar) is usually also used so as not to rely unduly on the nose ring for control. If the bull has horns, the lead rope may also be fastened around those and then passed down through the nose ring. Some shows require other cattle to be led with nose grips (bulldogs). Several methods exist for handling a bull with a ring installed. One method of leading a bull is to have one person on either side of the bull with both halter lead ropes through the ring, which prevents the bull from gaining pace and also from running into the handlers. Another practice is for one handler to use a rope and the other a bull-staff attached to the ring.

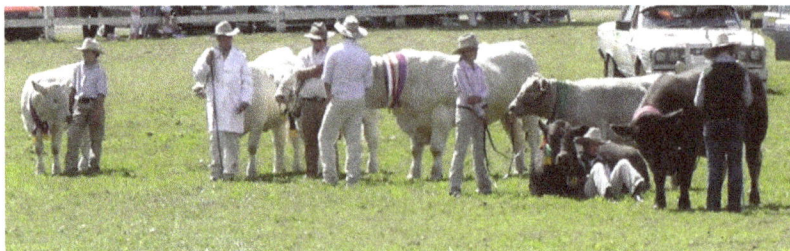
Charolais & Murray Grey bulls on parade with nose rings and a show lead ring

Bull handling on the Farm or Ranch

It is estimated that 42% of all livestock-related human fatalities are a result of bull attacks, and only about one in twenty victims of a bull attack survives. Dairy breed bulls are particularly dangerous and unpredictable; the hazards of bull handling are a significant cause of injury and death for dairy farmers in some parts of the United States. Most cattle breeders recognize the importance of looking after expensive bulls that are expected to improve herds and profits. Nonetheless, the dangers of bull handling, particularly from dairy bulls in close quarters, are regularly proven by the obituaries. Good bull management and safety practices require caution in handling beef and dairy bulls, and use of the nose ring and chain is a recommended precaution for modern farmers.

However, in many regions, particularly in the beef industry, bulls do not have nose rings unless they are to be exhibited and they are generally driven about as other cattle would be. Cows with young calves can be particularly dangerous if protecting their young, and cattle in general, including calves, steers and bullocks, do cause many serious human injuries and deaths.

Generally the use of both a ring and a halter, and management of the bull by two people, is the preferred method today for controlling the bull. Typically, a bull was led by a wooden staff with a steel end that snapped into the ring. A long rigid steel or wooden bull staff locked into the ring could also be used to push a bull out of a pen without requiring the handler to enter the pen for cleaning or feeding. Because of the risk that the bull may drive the staff into the handler if the bull misbehaves many handlers prefer to avoid their use nowadays. One current veterinary text still recommends the use of a staff in addition to the halter.

Many handlers rely on a nose ring to control a bull. But a ring in his nose is no good unless you have a bull staff and use it. A bull staff is a pole with a snap in the end that clips to the bull ring. Leading a bull with a staff gives you a lot more handling power as the bull can't get any closer to you than the length of the staff allows. Leading him only by a chain in the ring lets him run over you at will.

Most dairy or beef farms traditionally had at least one, if not several, bulls for breeding purposes. The handling of an aggressive, powerful animal was a practical issue with life-threatening consequences for the farmer. The need to move the bull in and out of his pen to cover cows exposed the farmer to serious jeopardy of life and limb. Being trampled, jammed against a wall or gored by a bull was one of the most frequent causes of death in the dairy industry prior to 1940. As suggested in one popular farming magazine, "Handle [the bull] with a staff and take no chances. The gentle bull, not the vicious one, most often kills or maims his keeper."

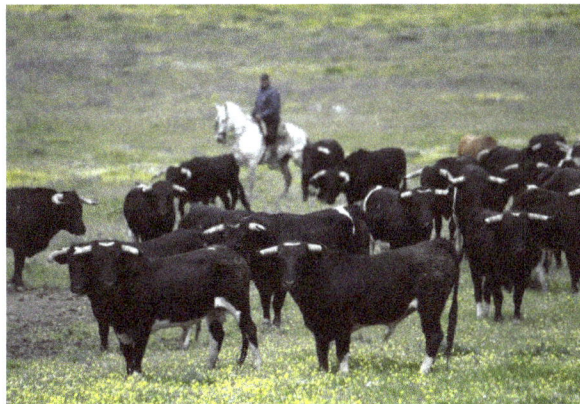
Bulls respond well to a good handler

When allowed outside his pen, the bull typically was kept in a halter connected by a strap snapped into the ring in his nose for ease of control. In the bull pen, the use of a ring connected by a cable to a fixed point was recommended as a means of controlling and securing the bull while allowing a degree of movement by the subject bull. If the pen was strong enough, the bull could be turned loose, and if needed, placed in a stanchion. Farmers who lacked an assistant, or a bull staff, had no choice but to adopt other means. Some farmers elected to move their bulls by tying a rope to the ring and tying the other end of the rope to a farm tractor, providing both motive power and a degree of protection from the angry bull. The efficacy of this technique is doubtful, and may depend on the size of the tractor and of the bull; one authority has "seen a bull lift the front end of a tractor like a toy". Others used dogs and horses. Not all farmers could afford specially designed and manufactured bull handling products, which were not readily available until the 1980s. The experimental improvisation of techniques for bull handling, as in many aspects of family farming, was a common practice.

Dysthanasia

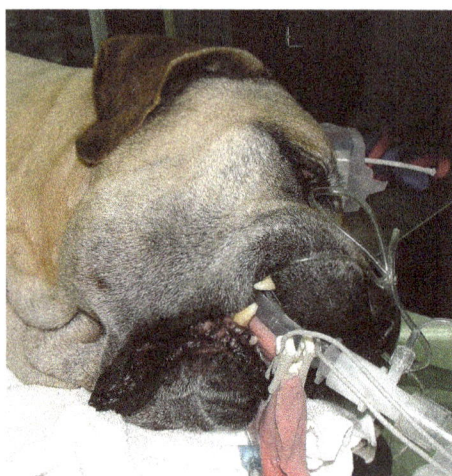

A geriatric mastiff with multiple tumors is being prepared for palliative surgery

Animal dysthanasia refers to the practice of prolonging the life of animals that are seriously or even terminally ill and that are potentially experiencing suffering. Animal dysthanasia is a recent concept, emerging from changes in the social perception of animals and from advances in veterinary care.

Context

Animal dysthanasia is particularly relevant in the context of small animal practice. For centuries, domestic animals in Western societies used to be mainly farm animals. With the industrialization process, humans become increasingly concentrated in urban areas, having preferential contact with companion animals, namely cats and dogs. While farm animals are widely seen as property, companion animals are perceived as family members with whom humans keep close bonds and develop strong emotional relationships.

At the same time, scientific advances in the field of veterinary medicine enable practitioners to reach accurate diagnoses faster and more reliably than before, allowing life-threatening illnesses to be identified in the early stages of their development. In addition, more advanced options of treatment are currently available which may sometimes be used to prolong the lives of animals as much as possible regardless of their quality.

The Companion Animal Euthanasia Training Academy (CAETA) defines dysthanasia differently. To align more closely with the current definition of euthanasia, the act of humanely terminating life, CAETA views dysthanasia as the opposite of euthanasia; an actual bad death event wherein the euthanasia went poorly. Any lack of care or suffering leading up to death is considered a lack of veterinary hospice support during the end of life.

Causes

Decision upon animal euthanasia often takes into account the relief of pain and suffering. Depending on how one defines the term, Animal dysthanasia occurs because there is no agreement upon the acceptable and recognizable endpoints of the lives of companion animals. This is due to several reasons. The keeper (guardian; owner) may wish to extend the animal's life because he rejects euthanasia as an acceptable solution. On the other hand, the veterinarian may have a scientific interest on studying the progress of a specific illness or even a financial interest in keeping the patient alive. If one defines dysthanasia as an actual bad death event, causes include use of improper euthanasia techniques or failure to render an animal free of pain or distress. Proper training in euthanasia procedures is ideal to reduce dysthanasia and subsequent suffering. The keeper and the veterinarian may also want to make use of all possible treatment resources before making the decision of euthanasia. Genuine belief on the animal's recovery and emotional attachment can also interfere in the decision-making process of euthanasia. Situations like these can be especially problematic in some veterinary specialities like small animal oncology where the course of the disease may be difficult to predict and the treatments themselves can cause severe distress.

Triple Tibial Osteotomy

The triple tibial osteotomy is a surgical procedure used to treat dogs that have completely or partially ruptured the cranial cruciate ligament in one or both of their stifles. The cranial cruciate ligament connects the femur with the tibia, which functions to stabilise the canine stifle joint from the forces put on it during exercise and weight bearing.

Stifle Joint in Dog

The stifle joint relies solely upon soft tissue structures for its integrity; thus it differs from an elbow or a hip joint that have a lot of parallel joint surfaces and an interlocking structure to the joints that give them inherent stability and an almost vacuum effect that keeps the joint surfaces together.

Along with the cranial cruciate ligament, the other soft tissue structures stabilising the stifle are the caudal cruciate ligament and the two menisci, all of which are intra-articular (within the joint), and the two collateral ligaments (external to the joint). Muscle tone through the quadriceps, hamstring and calf muscles play a significant role in the forces acting on the joint.

Cranial Cruciate Ligament

The cranial cruciate ligament is composed of two bands, a craniomedial band and a caudolateral band. It functions to stop cranial (anterior) movement of the tibia with respect to the femur, hyperextension of the stifle joint and internal rotation of the tibia. The cranial cruciate ligament is thought to be able to resist a force equivalent to four times the weight of the dog before it ruptures, but often the ligament is weakened by arthritis that is present in the joint. Arthritis infers inflammation of the joint; in this condition there is the production of a joint fluid that is less viscous and therefore less able to absorb shock than normal fluid. Joint fluid's other role is to provide nutrition to the cartilage and the cruciate ligaments. The situation is a little like a chicken-and-egg scenario: it is usually accepted that the cranial cruciate ligament ruptures because arthritis has caused the ligament to weaken because of poor joint fluid characteristics, but what causes the arthritis in the first place – a partial cruciate tear?

The situation is dissimilar to that seen in human athletes where overextension of the joint stretches the cranial cruciate ligament to failure, and replacement of the ligament with a fascial prosthesis has a good prognosis for return to full function.

Menisci

The menisci are the other intra-articular structures that help to stabilise the joint and help to distribute load evenly across the surfaces; these are crescent-shaped discs of cartilage facing each other from side to side across the joint. They are thicker at the outside and with a thin inner aspect and they also have nerve fibres that help to tell the brain how much load is getting transmitted through the joint. The medial (inside) meniscus is often damaged with a long-standing cruciate ligament rupture because it is firmly attached to the tibia and gets crushed during abnormal cranial movement of the tibia. The lateral (outside) meniscus is more firmly attached to the femur and does not get crushed.

Surgical Rationale

The triple tibial osteotomy was developed by a New Zealand veterinary orthopaedic specialist, Dr. Warrick Bruce, while he was working in Adelaide, South Australia. By changing the geometry of the forces of gravity and muscle contractions that act on the stifle during weight-bearing, it aims to neutralise the shear force that causes the cranial movement of the tibia with respect to the femur.

This shear force develops because the canine tibial plateau – the weight-bearing aspect of the joint – is sloped caudally (downwards towards the back of the joint)and there is an acute angle between the tibial plateau slope and the patellar ligament. In the triple tibial osteotomy procedure, the tibia has three osteotomies (cuts into the bone with a bone saw) performed upon it with the aim of realigning the tibial plateau slope so that it ultimately becomes aligned at right angles to the patellar ligament instead of sloping backwards. By achieving this, shear forces within the joint are neutralised and the joint is stable as the dog weight-bears.

The joint is not stable, however, when it is physically manipulated by attempting to move the tibia cranially. This contrasts with previous methods of cranial cruciate ligament repair which aimed to provide stability to the joint by replacing the ligament either with a fascial graft within the joint, or using a prosthesis made of nylon placed externally from the lateral fabella to a hole drilled in the tibial crest.

The triple tibial osteotomy has been developed as a hybrid of two previously available orthopaedic procedures, the tibial tuberosity advancement and the tibial plateau leveling osteotomy. The tibial tuberosity advancement neutralises shear force within the stifle by advancing the tibial tuberosity until the tibial plateau is at right angles to the patellar ligament. The tibial plateau leveling osteotomy neutralises shear force by rotating the tibial plateau so that it is approximately horizontal with respect to the long axis of the tibia. The triple tibial osteotomy combines both of these procedures and as such less radical changes than either are required.

Surgical Technique

The triple tibial osteotomy involves removing a horizontal small wedge of bone (average 16 degrees) halfway along a vertical osteotomy in the tibial tuberosity. Firstly by removing the wedge of bone, the tibial plateau is levelled. Secondly as the horizontal defect created by removing the wedge is closed down, the tibial tuberosity is itself advanced by several millimetres. This compares with an average of 20 degrees plateau levelling required for the tibial plateau leveling osteotomy and 9-12mm of tibial tuberosity advancement with the tibial tuberosity advancement.

Return to normal function is rapid, with most dogs having good use of the leg and a normal appearing gait within 3–4 months; long-term progression of arthritis is minimal.

Procedures in Sheep

Despite their gentle nature and capacity to suffer as any other animal, sheep aren't protected by the same laws as dogs and cats. 'Codes of Practice' side-step the rules, allowing farmers to cut bits and pieces off young lambs without even providing them pain relief.

Tail Docking

Like puppies, lambs are born with a long tail. But most lambs are put in a restraint device and have their tail cut off (like tail docking: to reduce soiling and the risk of flystrike). When lambs are less than 6 months old, this practice can be done without anything to dull the pain. Often lambs are also mulesed at the same time.

A hot blade or sharp knife is used to cut through the muscle and bone of the lamb's tail. On some farms, lambs will instead have a rubber ring tightened around their tail so that it will wither and drop off.

If a lamb's tail is cut too short, they are at higher risk of suffering from serious health complications, such as rectal prolapse.

Mulesing

Young lambs often have the skin around their buttocks and the base of their tail cut off with a pair of metal shears (to reduce soiling and the risk of flystrike). This painful practice, called mulesing, has been banned in New Zealand for cruelty, but sadly can still legally be performed in Australia without any pain relief.

The large, open wound created by mulesing can take many weeks to heal. During this time, lambs are at added risk of infection and flystrike.

While mulesing is inflicted on lambs to reduce flystrike, several other less invasive and much less painful solutions exist. In 2010, the leaders of the Australian wool industry backed down on a commitment to phase out mulesing in favour of more humane alternatives. In 2016, wool industry leaders would not even support mandatory use of pain relief for mulesed lambs (let alone start a phase-out of mulesing), so sadly millions of lambs in Australia are continuing to undergo this cruel surgery, many with no pain relief whatsoever.

Castration

Male lambs usually have to endure both castration and tail docking (and sometimes mulesing) at the same time. When these procedures are carried out by unskilled people, the risk of greater injury, and infection is even more significant.

Shearing

Shearing is not only stressful for sheep who are inherently fearful of human handling but rough treatment in the shearing shed also puts them at risk of injury. Sheep are often cut by the sharp shearing blades, and when they suffer larger wounds, it is considered acceptable industry practice to stitch them up without providing any pain relief. As with those who carry out other painful, invasive procedures, there is currently no requirement for shearers to undergo formal training and accreditation.

Invasive Breeding Procedures

Female sheep are also often forced to endure invasive procedures. In one common breeding procedure, called laparoscopic artificial insemination, a long metal rod is poked through the ewe's abdomen to insert semen into her uterus. This invasive procedure can be done without pain relief.

References

- Muir, William W.; Hubbell, John A. E. (1995). Handbook of Veterinary Anesthesia (2nd ed.). Mosby. ISBN 0-8016-7656-8

- What-is-declawing: drkindklaws.com, Retrieved 14 March, 2019

- Villeda, Ray (2014-04-29). "Fort Worth Vet Accused of Keeping Dog Alive for Transfusions | NBC 5 Dallas-Fort Worth". Nbcdfw.com. Retrieved 2016-01-03

- Primary Industries Ministerial Council (2006). The Sheep - Second Edition. Model Code of Practice for the Welfare of Animals. CSIRO Publishing. ISBN 0-643-09357-5. Retrieved 2007-01-09

- Sheep-painful-procedures, issues: animalsaustralia.org, Retrieved 25 January, 2019

- Rollin BE (2006) "Euthanasia and quality of life", Journal American Veterinary Medical Association, 228(7): 1014-1016

5
Veterinary Vaccines and Drugs

Veterinary vaccines and drugs play a major role in promoting animal health and reducing animal suffering. Some of the common veterinary vaccines are clostridial vaccine, DA2PPC vaccine and rabies vaccine. There are a number of drugs which are used to treat different ailments in animals. A few of them are acepromazine, boldenone and butorphanol. The diverse applications of these drugs and vaccines have been thoroughly discussed in this chapter.

Veterinary Vaccines

Vaccination has long been an effective way to reduce disease burden in pets and farm animals, and is a key tool in maintaining animal health and welfare. Vaccines continue to play an increasingly vital role in preventative health and disease control programmes in animals. Innovative research and the development of safe, effective and quality vaccines means that our pets and farm animals continue to benefit from vital medicines that prevent or alleviate clinical signs of disease.

All those who care for animals, including pet owners and farmers have a duty to protect the health and welfare of animals under their care. However, animals, like people, are susceptible to a wide range of diseases caused by viruses, bacteria, fungi and parasites. Vaccines are available for many of these diseases, making them preventable or mitigating the losses or long term consequences of disease. This is particularly important for those diseases which have complex, limited or no treatment options available. Therefore, we should prioritise preventing disease or minimising the clinical signs of disease in the first instance to protect the health and welfare of animals: the old adage of 'prevention is better than cure'.

Reassuringly, effective vaccines are available for many important animal diseases. Some of these diseases are endemic, meaning they are normally found in the UK e.g. Canine Parvovirus in dogs, or they may be exotic, meaning that they are not normally found in the UK. However they may still pose a risk for entry to the UK e.g. Bluetongue in sheep and cattle or Rabies from travelling pets. For many years, the animal medicines sector has continued to invest in the research and development of veterinary vaccines to tackle these endemic and exotic diseases. One of the greatest achievements in veterinary medicine in modern times has been the global eradication of a devastating disease of livestock – Rinderpest in 2011, for which vaccination played a central role.

Even though many diseases are successfully controlled with vaccination, despite best efforts, effective vaccines can sometimes prove technically very difficult to develop. This is due to the complex nature of vaccine development and the inherent characteristics of some pathogens. Ongoing investment in research and development aims to tackle these challenges and make available more vaccines to maintain animal health and welfare. Indeed, vaccines are often updated to include and protect against new strains as diseases evolve. The challenge in developing new vaccines reminds us that vaccines are part of a wider range of animal medicines – that together protect and treat our companion and farm animals.

Regulation and Veterinary Vaccines

All authorised veterinary medicines, including vaccines available in the UK, must undergo a strict regulatory approval process, before they gain a Marketing Authorisation (MA) (commonly called a product licence) for sale and supply. Stringent evaluation, by independent regulatory authorities, the Veterinary Medicines Directorate (VMD) in the UK and the European Medicines Agency (EMA) in the EU, ensure that each authorised vaccine meets the required high standards of safety, efficacy and quality.

In the UK, animal vaccines can be classified based on their authorised supply route, and are either POM-V (prescription only medicines – through a veterinary surgeon) or, in the case of some farm animal vaccines, POM-VPS (Prescription Only Medicine – Veterinary Surgeon, Pharmacist, Suitably Qualified Person (SQP)).

After vaccines are licensed and used in animals, their continued efficacy and safety is monitored through a surveillance system whereby any adverse events can be reported to Market Authorisation Holder (MAH) of the vaccine or to the VMD. This ensures that there is an opportunity for continual monitoring and, if necessary, further improvement in the safety of these medicines.

Key Concepts: Vaccines and Vaccination

Vaccines have a long and successful history of preventing and controlling disease. The veterinary vaccines available today represent years of innovative research and meet many of the disease threats faced by pets and farm animals in the UK today.

Vaccines work by stimulating an immune response in an animal without causing the disease itself. When healthy animals are vaccinated, their own immune system responds to the vaccine and can remember the infectious agent to which the animal is vaccinated. This means, if appropriately vaccinated animals are then exposed to the pathogen against which they have been vaccinated, they can expect a level of protection from disease.

The main types of vaccines available can be categorised as modified-live (attenuated), inactivated and recombinant:

- Modified-live (attenuated): A vaccine that contains an intact but weakened pathogen which stimulates an immune response but does not cause clinical disease.

- Inactivated (killed): A vaccine that contains a completely inactivated pathogen, which is no longer infectious. These vaccines often contain an adjuvant, which is a compound added to help improve the protective immune response.

- Recombinant: A vaccine that is produced using genetic engineering technology and using specific genetic material from a pathogen to produce proteins which will stimulate an immune response when the animal is vaccinated.

- Toxoid: A vaccine that is based on inactivated toxins produced by pathogens. These vaccines stimulate immunity and protect the animal against these toxins.

Research and innovation has also resulted in the development of novel and more sophisticated technologies such as marker vaccines. Typically, when animals are vaccinated they produce an immune response that resembles that of a natural infection. It can then be difficult when testing animals to determine if they have been naturally infected or if they have been vaccinated. An example is the farm animal marker vaccine for Infectious Bovine Rhinotracheitis (IBR) – a highly contagious respiratory disease in cattle.

Irrespective of the type of vaccine used, an animal should be in good health at the time of vaccination – as a properly functioning immune system is needed to stimulate a good immune response and develop an effective level of protection. Initially a primary vaccination course should be completed and depending on the vaccine type and the species of animal, it may be necessary to follow up with booster vaccinations at intervals based on veterinary advice and the characteristics of the vaccine, to maintain protective immunity throughout the animals' lifetime.

There is no 'one size fits all' when vaccinating animals and vaccination protocols should be tailored, based on veterinary consultation, for individual pets or groups of farm animals. This is because animals are exposed to a range of different risk factors related to their age, lifestyle, prevailing disease threats and travel/movement. These factors should be discussed with the vet to decide on the most appropriate choice of vaccine and vaccination protocol. For some farm animal vaccines, appropriate advice can also be sought from an SQP.

Another important concept in vaccination is that of 'herd immunity'. Herd immunity is the protection offered to a wider community of animals, pets or farm animals, when a sufficiently high proportion of individual animals are vaccinated, reducing the prevalence of disease and numbers of susceptible individuals in an area. An unfortunate example of what can happen when herd immunity diminishes were the outbreaks of measles in the UK in recent years, which are thought to be due to reduced numbers of children being vaccinated.

Public health can also be protected through vaccination and a good example of this is the requirement for cats, dogs and ferrets to have a valid rabies vaccination before entering or returning to the UK from abroad. Vaccination plays a key role in protecting animals and people in the UK from the threat of rabies, which is still one of the most deadly zoonoses (meaning diseases which can be passed from animals to humans).

Vaccination can also help support the responsible use of antibiotics by preventing disease or reducing clinical signs so that fewer veterinary medicine treatments are needed. Although antibiotics are only useful for bacterial infections, there are many cases where farm animals and pets succumb to viral disease in the first instance, which then leads to a subsequent secondary bacterial infection that may need treatment with antibiotics. So vaccinating for both bacterial and viral disease can help to preserve the future effectiveness of antibiotics.

Companion Animal Vaccination

The mainstay of protecting our pets from a wide range of diseases, many of which are very difficult or impossible to treat, is through vaccination. Our pets enjoy the protection from disease despite the risks they face every day from the environment, from travelling and from direct and indirect contact with unvaccinated or diseased animals. As every pet is faced with different risk factors, it is very important to discuss these with the vet, so the most appropriate vaccinations are provided. The information about the different vaccines is publically available, provided in the Summary of Product Characteristics (SPC) associated with each individual UK authorised vaccine. As recommended by the VMD, the vet should take the SPC and specific risk factors associated with each animal into account when they are developing a suitable vaccination schedule.

Feline Vaccination

Many of the most important diseases in cats can be prevented, controlled or alleviated through effective vaccination. These include:

- Feline Panleukopenia/Infectious Enteritis (Feline Panleukopenia or Parvovirus, FPV)

- Feline Rhinotracheitis (Feline Herpesvirus, FHV)

- Feline Calicivirus (FCV)

- Feline Leukaemia Virus (FeLV)

- Chlamydophila felis

- Feline Rabies.

In 2015, the European Advisory Board on Cat Diseases (ABCD) produced updated best practice vaccination guidelines for indoor and outdoor cats, rescue shelter cats and breeding catteries. These guidelines recommend that 'core' vaccines should be administered to all cats (FPV, FHV, FCV) and 'non-core' are recommended only for cats at risk of specific infection. Additionally, 'circumstantial' vaccines are needed in specific circumstances such as Rabies vaccination for cats travelling in and out of the UK – often referred to as the PETS travel scheme. The ABCD also provide recommendations on vaccination schedules for the primary vaccination course and subsequent boosters, which take into consideration the type of vaccine product and vaccination history.

Canine Vaccination

The UK veterinary medicines regulator, the VMD, have published a position paper on authorised vaccination schedules for dogs including core and non-core vaccines. The important canine diseases, for which vaccines are available, include:

- Canine Distemper Virus (CDV)

- Canine Parvovirus (CPV)

- Canine Adenovirus (CAV)

- Canine Leptospira

- Canine parainfluenza virus (CPi)

- Bordetella bronchiseptica

- Canine Rabies.

The core canine UK vaccines include CDV, CAV and CPV – these protect dogs from severe life threating viruses, whilst canine leptospira, CPi and Bordetella bronchiseptica for animals who are at risk due to their geographical location, local environment or lifestyle and are considered non-core. Other UK vaccines authorised for use in dogs in Canine Herpes and Canine Coronavirus (Canine Enteric Coronavirus, CECOV).

Farm Animal Vaccination

Farm animals are represented by a variety of different species, from cattle, sheep, pigs and poultry to farmed fish. This means there is a correspondingly diverse range of potential disease threats and vaccines available to protect farm animals.

Disease outbreaks can occur when new stock are brought in to replenish the herd or flock, or when an animal becomes ill and disease may spread within susceptible animals housed or grouped together. Taken together, the challenges faced by farm animals means there is an ongoing requirement for effective, safe, quality vaccines – not only for the endemic diseases, but also during periods of exotic disease threat.

A good example of vaccines used on farm as part of an endemic disease control programme in the UK is that of Bovine Viral Diarrhoea (BVD) in cattle. An example of an exotic disease threat faced by cattle and sheep is Bluetongue, for which vaccination is the effective way to help prevent the spread of disease.

In aquaculture too the innovative development of vaccine products supports fish health and welfare and the productivity of an important and growing sector in the UK.

Farm animal vaccination strategies are developed as part of preventative farm health plans, which aim to vaccinate based on individual farm risk for particular diseases. Species-specific guidelines on responsible use of vaccines and vaccination are produced by RUMA (Responsible Use of Medicines in Agriculture Alliance).

The production of safe, affordable food from healthy animals is an increasing priority in a growing global population. Farmers are meeting this need by embracing animal medicine innovation to improve health and welfare and prevent losses where possible. The use of vaccines on farm is also becoming increasingly important at a time when farmers and vets are refining and improving their responsible use of antibiotics.

Equine Vaccination

Horses as companion animals, athletes and breeding stock are exposed to varied disease threats depending on their unique circumstances. Risk factors including travelling to other geographical regions and mixing with unvaccinated horses are also very important.

Important equines vaccines include Equine Influenza, Tetanus, Equine Herpes Virus 1 and 4 (EHV-1 and EHV-4). Other vaccines that are authorised for use in horses in the UK include those for equine viral arteritis, equine rotavirus, Streptococcus equi equi and West Nile Virus. Depending on the lifestyle and use of the horse specific vaccinations are recommended. Vaccination of all horses is recommended for equine tetanus, which can be fatal and equine influenza, which is a contagious viral respiratory disease. Many equestrian organisations and all racecourse premises require mandatory vaccination for equine influenza. Regular EHV vaccination is important for breeding stock, particularly in stud farms, to help reduce reproductive losses and respiratory disease.

Clostridial Vaccine

A clostridial vaccine is a vaccine for sheep that protects against diseases caused by toxins produced by an infection with one or more *Clostridium* bacteria. Clostridial vaccines are often administered to pregnant ewes a few weeks before they are due to give birth, in order to give passive immunity to their lambs. Clostridial bacteria multiply rapidly in infected sheep, and produce large amounts of toxin which can cause the sheep to die within hours.

Clostridial vaccines can contain anti-toxins to one or more endotoxins produced by the following bacteria:

- Clostridium chauvoei
- Clostridium haemolyticum
- Clostridium novyi
- Clostridium perfringens
- Clostridium septicum
- Clostridium sordellii
- Clostridium tetani.

Clostridial vaccines which protect sheep against multiple clostridial diseases have been available since the 1950s.

DA2PPC Vaccine

DA2PP is a multivalent vaccine for dogs that protects against the viruses indicated by the alphanumeric characters forming the acronym: D for canine distemper, A2 for canine adenovirus type 2, which offers cross-protection to canine adenovirus type 1 (the more pathogenic of the two strains), the first P for canine parvovirus, and the second P for parainfluenza. Because infectious canine hepatitis is another name for canine adenovirus type 1, an H is sometimes used instead of A. In DA2PPC, the C indicates canine coronavirus.

This vaccine is usually given to puppies at 8 weeks of age, followed by 12 weeks of age, and then 16 weeks of age. This vaccine is given again at 1 year of age and then annually, or every 3 years. Some veterinarians' recommended vaccine schedules may differ from this.

DA2PPC does not include *Bordetella*. But the combination of *Bordetella* with DA2PPC prevents kennel cough, by preventing adenovirus, distemper, parainfluenza, *and Bordetella*.

For Distemper

While the DA2PPC vaccine also protects against parainfluenza, parvovirus, adenovirus, and canine coronavirus, it most importantly protects against the debilitating and deadly disease canine distemper, an often fatal viral illness that causes neurologic dysfunction, pneumonia, nonspecific systemic symptoms such as fever and fatigue, and weight loss, as well as upper respiratory symptoms and diarrhea, poor appetite, and vomiting. There is no antiviral drug effective against the canine distemper virus. Treatment is supportive and consists of antibiotics to prevent secondary infections, anticonvulsants for seizures, and intravenus fluids to prevent dehydration. Given the lethality of distemper and the relative rarity of side effects from the vaccine, all reputable veterinarians recommend the DA2PPC vaccine. Also, even if the dog owner is not concerned about adenovirus, coronavirus, parvovirus, or parainfluenza, they should vaccinate their dogs to protect them against distemper.

DHPP, DAPP, DA2PP, and DAPPC are not the same. The names are often used interchangeably but they are different. Distemper, adenovirus type 1 (thus hepatitis), parainfluenza, and parvovirus are covered by all 4. DHPP covers adenovirus type 1 and may or may not cover adenovirus type 2. And only DAPPC covers coronavirus. DAPP or DA2PP are the most commonly used.

Rabies Vaccine

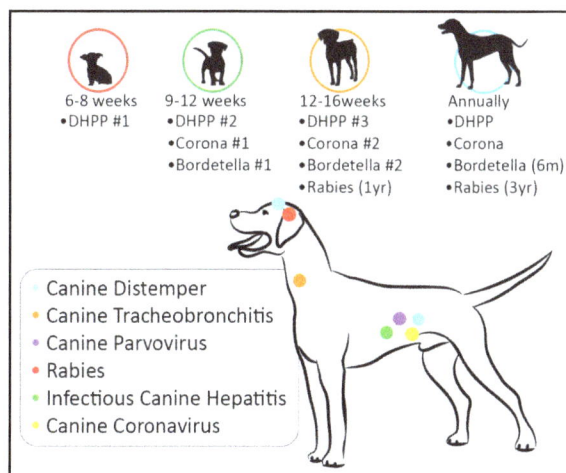

Rabies vaccination timeline for pets

Rabies vaccines come in several different forms; some are good for one year, while others are good for three years. All Rabies vaccines for dogs, and some rabies vaccines for cats are adjuvanted (an adjuvant is an agent added to a vaccine to help stimulate the immune system). An adjuvant helps a pet create a more robust immune response to a vaccine. Whether a vaccine is good for one year or three depends on the presence of an adjuvant as well as the nature of the studies run by the vaccine companies. When using an adjuvanted vaccine approved for 3 years, there is no difference as far as local laws are concerned. What makes your pet's rabies vaccination good for one year or three years is determined by two things:

- The animal's age and rabies vaccine history

- If the state and municipal laws require annual vaccinations for rabies.

Dogs and cats are first vaccinated for rabies between 3 and 6 months of age. They need a booster one year from that date. They are then generally vaccinated every three years, although some states still require annual rabies vaccinations for dogs and/or cats.

General Confusion about Vaccinations

There have been lots of discussions (and confusion) about cat and dog vaccinations. How often, what vaccinations are really necessary, do risks outweigh benefits, and so on. The standard of care for decades was to vaccinate dogs and cats annually for several common diseases, without much "choice" about specific vaccinations or schedules. The recommendation from the American Animal Hospital Association (AAHA) and most veterinarians and is to give core vaccines (vaccines that are considered necessary for every dog or cat) every three years, with careful selection of the vaccines needed for each specific pet. Most lifestyle vaccines (vaccines that are given on a case by case basis based on a pet's lifestyle) still need to be given every year due to the nature of those specific diseases.

Rabies the Disease vs. Rabies the Vaccine

The one exception to vaccine "choice" is the rabies vaccine. It is the only vaccination required by law in the United States, as rabies is a fatal disease. It is also a zoonotic disease, meaning it may be transmitted from animals to humans. There is no cure for rabies. Vaccinating for rabies will help an animal mount an immune system response to protect against rabies, but it isn't a curative treatment.

How Long do Vaccines Offer Protection?

This is the big question. There isn't one answer. How long a vaccine, rabies or otherwise, is "good" for, in terms of actual disease protection is still debated. The vaccine, the health of the individual and their immune system, the disease agents, all of these factors come into play.

Titers have been touted as a way to measure protection, but this is still a topic under discussion. A titer is a blood test that measures antibody levels; the immune system's reminder of previous exposure to an infectious agent or vaccine. This is not necessarily a measure of how the body will react to a new challenge with the disease agent. Titers aren't harmful to run and do provide some information. There is a cost involved to run these test(s). In addition, rabies titers do not replace the legal need to get an updated Rabies vaccine for your pet in accordance with your local laws. Speak with your veterinarian for their opinion and to discuss if this is a useful protocol for your pet.

Adjuvanted vs. Non-Adjuvanted Vaccines

Thanks to a 1991 letter to the editor in the Journal of the American Veterinary Medical Association, a possible connection to adjuvanted rabies vaccines and sarcomas in cats was raised. This discussion led to the formation of the Vaccine-Associated Feline Sarcoma Task Force to tabulate and track vaccination data.

As a result of these studies, non-adjuvanted vaccines are now available for cats. These vaccines come in one year and three year forms.

From the VAFSTF: "While a specific cause has not been established, it is thought that inflammatory processes related to administration of injectable products can lead to the formation of sarcomas. The role of adjuvants (including those containing aluminum) and local inflammation in the pathogenesis of FISS is not clear. (An adjuvant is a substance added to the vaccine to increase the effectiveness of the component antigens, such as killed microorganisms in an induction of an immune response.)"

From UC Davis College of Veterinary Medicine: "We currently stock and suggest the use of the recombinant rabies vaccine, because there is some evidence that it is associated with a decreased risk of sarcoma formation."

Vaccine requirements for each pet and geographic location are different. Please speak to your veterinarian about the best vaccination protocol for your specific pet(s), location, and lifestyle.

Vaccination of Cattle

Brucella abortus is a bacterium that causes brucellosis in cattle. B. abortus RB51 is a strain of this bacterium developed specifically for immunization of cattle against brucellosis to allow serological differentiation between naturally infected and vaccinated animals.

Accidental human exposure to RB51, though uncommon, has resulted in development of symptoms consistent with brucellosis. Exposures have included needle sticks, eye and wound splashes, and contact with infected material.

Other vaccines, such as Brucella abortus S19 for cattle and B. melitensis Rev-1 for sheep and goats, can also cause infection in humans.

Veterinarians and other medical staff performing immunizations in cattle should be aware of the risks and what to do when an exposure occurs. S19 and Rev-1 exposures should follow the same assessment guidance as for RB51. Serological monitoring is available for S19 and Rev-1 exposures.

Rabbit Vaccination

Protecting the health and welfare of pet rabbits involves taking a proactive approach to preventative healthcare. Vaccination of pet rabbits is an important part of this approach and is widely recommended to protect rabbits from two very serious viral infectious diseases – myxomatosis and rabbit haemorrhagic disease. All veterinary medicines authorised for use in the UK, including rabbit vaccines against these two diseases, have met high standards of quality, safety and efficacy as assessed by an independent veterinary regulator.

There are an estimated 0.6 million pet rabbits in the UK. All of these rabbits, just like cats and dogs, are susceptible to infectious diseases that have a serious effect on their health and welfare. In some cases infection will result in rabbits needing prolonged intensive care treatment and in many cases the most serious viral diseases of rabbits are fatal.

Two very important viral rabbit diseases are myxomatosis and rabbit haemorrhagic disease (RHD):

- Myxomatosis is a disease to which all breeds of domesticated, as well as wild, rabbits are at risk. It is typically spread by blood sucking insects including rabbit fleas, mosquitos and mites and by direct contact with infected rabbits. All rabbits are at potential risk of infection as the disease can be carried over distances by insects, which can then come into contact with indoor as well as outdoor rabbits. Signs of the disease include swellings, including the head/face/ears, which can cause blindness and affect their ability to feed and drink. The disease is frequently fatal and so vaccination, along with flea control, good husbandry and stress reduction, is recommended.

- Rabbit haemorrhagic disease (RHD), also known as Viral Haemorrhagic Disease (VHD) is another very serious infectious disease of rabbits. All rabbits are again at potential risk as it is spread by both direct and indirect contact with infected rabbits. Indirect transfer can occur via people and their clothing, through contaminated hutches and bedding, as well as insect vectors such as fleas and flies. The disease is endemic in wild rabbits in the UK. Signs of infection in rabbits include being depressed or collapsed, breathing difficulties, convulsions, a fever and bleeding from the nose. Death can occur very rapidly, within 12-36 hours of a fever, and mortality rates can be extremely high. Unfortunately, rabbits are often found dead. More recently, another new variant of RHD has emerged (RHD-2) and owners should be aware that following a consultation with their vet, rabbits may also need further vaccination against this strain.

Vaccinating to protect rabbits against these deadly diseases therefore makes good sense and the benefits are clearly evident in terms of reducing rabbit suffering and death and alleviating owner distress.

Vaccine Development, Approval and Monitoring

Vaccine research and development requires years of investment and expertise from veterinary scientists to produce suitable vaccines that meet high standards of safety, quality and efficacy as assessed and approved by independent regulators, which are the Veterinary Medicines Directorate (VMD) in UK and the European Medicines Agency (EMA) in the EU. Even after a vaccine is approved and becomes available for pets, animal medicine companies continue to support the safety and efficacy of their vaccines through a process of pharmacovigilance. Pharmacovigilance means vets and owners can report any suspected adverse reactions, which must then be reviewed by animal medicine companies and the VMD. Serious adverse reactions are very rare. Nevertheless, ongoing assessment helps to reduce these rare events even further. These responsibilities are taken seriously by animal medicines companies who continue to work and ensure that vaccines remain safe and effective into the future.

Rabbit Vaccines and Vaccination

Vaccines are available for the two main diseases of pet rabbits in the UK, namely myxomatosis and rabbit haemorrhagic disease (RHD) type 1 and type 2.

It is widely recommended that pet rabbits are vaccinated against these serious viral diseases as part of a preventative healthcare plan.

As the characteristics of individual vaccines can differ, the timings for vaccination and the frequency of booster vaccinations will depend on factors such as the duration of immunity from specific vaccines.

The benefits of vaccination can be exerted beyond the protection of individual rabbits. The prevalence of disease in regional communities can also be reduced by decreasing the overall numbers of susceptible rabbits that have not been vaccinated. When a high proportion of rabbits in the community are vaccinated the protection offered is called 'herd immunity'.

A vaccination appointment not only helps to protect your animal against infectious diseases, it also enables pet owners to discuss any concerns with their veterinary surgeon and allows the vet to perform a full health examination and diagnose any issues that need to be addressed, nipping potential problems in the bud.

We have a legal and moral responsibility to protect the animals in our care from pain, suffering and disease. Responsible rabbit ownership includes regular veterinary health visits and ensuring preventative steps are taken to avoid the negative welfare consequences of ill health. Working with vets, owners can proactively take steps to ensure reasonable preventative measures are taken to protect the health and welfare of their pet rabbits.

Veterinary Drugs

Veterinary drugs are used to cure and prevent diseases in animals, including animals used for food production. Veterinary drugs are given to animals via feed or drinking water, or by injection. The use of veterinary drugs may result in residues of these drugs in animal products like milk, eggs and meat. A lot of countries have established legal limits for residues of veterinary drugs in food.

Acepromazine

Acepromazine maleate is a phenothiazine derivative that is used as a neuroleptic agent in veterinary medicine. It is a commonly used tranquilizer for dogs, cats, and horses. Phenothiazines decrease dopamine levels and depress some portions of the reticular activating system. Acepromazine is metabolized by the liver and excreted in the urine.

In addition to tranquilization, acepromazine has multiple other important systemic effects including anti-cholinergic, anti-emetic, antispasmodic, antihistaminic, and alpha-adrenergic blocking properties. Acepromazine causes hypotension due to decreased vasomotor tone. It may change heart and respiratory rate and thermoregulatory ability allowing for either hypo- or hyper-thermia.

Acepromazine may be given intramuscularly, intravenously, or orally. It provides no analgesia and the tranquilizing effect of the drug can be overcome unexpectedly, particularly by sensory stimulation. Acepromazine usually is less effective if given after the animal is excited. There is a great deal of individual variability in the response to acepromazine and despite being a very commonly used medication there are important species and even breed differences in response to acepromazine that need to be taken into consideration.

Dogs and Cats

Acepromazine is one of the most commonly used tranquilizers for dogs and cats. It decreases anxiety, causes central nervous system depression, and a drop in blood pressure and heart rate. It may be used in conjunction with atropine as a pre-operative medication for anxiety and for its antidysrhythmic effects. Oral acepromazine may be prescribed to prevent motion sickness, to temporarily reduce itching and scratching due to allergies, or prior to office visits, nail trimming, or grooming appointments if the animal is too fractious to handle safely without sedation. Some veterinarians are reluctant to prescribe acepromazine for travel anxiety when the animal may be exposed to temperature extremes, such as during plane travel or when there may be limited access to veterinary care. Other drugs used for travel anxiety/motion sickness include meclizine, diphenhydramine, and diazepam. Occasionally, animals (particularly cats) may have a paradoxical response to acepromazine and become excited or aggressive.

Horses

Acepromazine is one of the most commonly used tranquilizers for horses. It may be used alone or in combination with other sedative drugs such as xylazine, detomidine, or butorphanol. Because acepromazine lowers blood pressure by dilating small blood-vessels, it sometimes is prescribed in the early treatment of laminitis in order to diminish vasospasm, and possibly to improve circulation within the hoof.

Acepromazine is also used in horses that are prone to exertional rhabdomyolysis both as a preventive and as a part of the treatment due to its vasodilatory properties. When acepromazine is used to treat more severe cases of exertional rhabdomyolysis, intravenous fluids may be desirable to increase hydration and to support renal function.

Onset of action of acepromazine varies with route of administration; oral acepromazine may take 30 minutes to one hour. The effects of acepromazine will last from one to four hours, but this varies significantly with dose and among individual horses. Acepromazine is a prohibited substance in most sanctioned competition. Oral administration or long-term, repeated dosing may increase detection time.

Side Effects

- Common: Acepromazine will cause hypotension, decreased respiratory rate, and bradycardia. Dogs are particularly sensitive to cardiovascular side-effects but cardiovascular collapse also has occurred in cats. Sudden collapse, decreased or absent pulse and breathing, pale gums, and unconsciousness may occur in some animals.

- Rare: Fatal interactions with anesthetics have been reported.

- Acepromazine will cause a dose-dependent decrease in hematocrit in both dogs and horses.

This effect occurs within 30 minutes of administration and may last for 12 hours or more. The hematocrit in horses may decrease by as much as 50%.

- Penile paralysis is a rare but recognized adverse side-effect of acepromazine use in the horse. This drug should be avoided in breeding stallions.

Precautions

- Acepromazine lowers blood pressure. It should not be used in animals that are dehydrated, anemic, or in shock.

- Acepromazine should be avoided or used with extreme caution in older animals or those with liver disease, heart disease, injury, or debilitation. If it is used in these animals, it should be given in very small doses. In some older animals, a very small dose can have a marked and very prolonged effect.

- Acepromazine should not be used in animals with a history of epilepsy, those prone to seizures, or those receiving a myelogram because it may lower the seizure threshold.

- Acepromazine should not be used in animals with tetanus or strychnine poisoning.

- Acepromazine should be avoided in pregnancy or lactation. It should be avoided or used with extreme caution in young animals due to its effects on an animal's ability to thermo regulate.

- Dogs: Giant breeds and greyhounds may be extremely sensitive to acepromazine, while terriers may require higher doses. Brachycephalic breeds, especially Boxers, are particularly prone to cardiovascular side-effects (drop in blood pressure and slow heart-rate). Acepromazine should be avoided or used with great caution in these breeds.

- Horses: Draft-horse breeds are especially sensitive to most sedatives including acepromazine. Pony breeds do not appear to differ from horses in their responses to acepromazine.

Drug Interactions

- Animals receiving acepromazine will require lower doses of barbiturates, narcotics and other anesthetics. These combinations increase central nervous system depression.

- Antidiarrheal mixtures like Kaopectate and Pepto-Bismol or antacids decrease the absorption of oral acepromazine.

- Acepromazine should not be used within one month of deworming with organophosphate compounds.

- Quinidine, epinephrine, propanolol, procaine hydrochloride, and phenytoin all have been shown to have significant drug-interactions with phenothiazines.

Overdose

- Overdose will cause excessive sedation, slow respiratory and heart rate, pale gums, unsteady gait, poor coordination, and inability to stand. It also may cause sudden collapse, unconsciousness, seizures, and death.

- Oral overdose should be treated by emptying the stomach along with monitoring and other supportive care.

- Phenylephrine and norepinephrine are the drugs-of-choice to treat acepromazine-induced hypotension. Barbiturates or diazepam may be used to treat seizures associated with overdose.

Boldenone

Boldenone undecylenate, or boldenone undecenoate, sold under the brand names Equipoise and Parenabol among others, is an androgen and anabolic steroid (AAS) medication which is used in veterinary medicine, mainly in horses. It was formerly used in humans as well. It is given by injection into muscle.

Side effects of boldenone undecylenate include symptoms of masculinization like acne, increased hair growth, voice changes, and increased sexual desire. The drug is a synthetic androgen and anabolic steroid and hence is an agonist of the androgen receptor (AR), the biological target of androgens like testosterone and dihydrotestosterone (DHT). It has strong anabolic effects and moderate androgenic effects, weak estrogenic effects, and no risk of liver damage. Boldenone undecylenate is an androgen ester and a long-lasting prodrug of boldenone in the body.

Boldenone undecylenate was introduced for medical use in the 1960s. In addition to its medical use, boldenone undecylenate is used to improve physique and performance. The drug is a controlled substance in many countries and so non-medical use is generally illicit. It remains marketed for veterinary use in Australia and the United States.

Uses

Veterinary: Boldenone undecylenate is used in veterinary medicine, mainly in horses.

Clinical: Boldenone undecylenate was formerly used in clinical medicine in humans, but was discontinued.

Pharmacology

Pharmacodynamics

Boldenone undecylenate is a prodrug of boldenone, and hence is an agonist of the androgen receptor. Boldenone has strong anabolic effects and moderate androgenic effects. It also has low estrogenic activity and has little or no progestogenic activity. In relation to the fact that it is not 17α-alkylated, boldenone and boldenone undecylenate have little or no risk of hepatotoxicity.

Pharmacokinetics

Boldenone undecylenate is a prodrug of boldenone. When administered via intramuscular injection, a depot is formed from which boldenone undecylenate is slowly released into the body and then transformed into boldenone. Boldenone undecylenate is reported to possess a biological half-life of 14 days when administered by intramuscular injection. Boldenone is a substrate for 5α-reductase and may be converted by this enzyme into 1-testosterone (δ^1-dihydrotestosterone, δ^1-DHT, dihydroboldenone) in tissues that express it such as the skin, hair follicles, and prostate gland. However, its affinity for this enzyme is said to be extremely low.

Chemistry

Boldenone undecylenate, or boldenone 17β-undec-10-enoate, is a synthetic androstane steroid and a derivative of testosterone. It is the C17β undecylenate (undecenoate) ester of boldenone (δ^1-testosterone, 1-dehydrotestosterone, or androsta-1,4-dien-17β-ol-3-one), which itself is the C1 dehydrogenated analogue of testosterone and a naturally occurring androgen found in the scent gland of *Ilybius fenestratus* (a species of aquatic beetle). Boldenone is the non-17α-alkylated variant of metandienone (17α-methyl-δ^1-testosterone). An AAS related to boldenone undecylenate is quinbolone (δ^1-testosterone 17β-cyclopentenyl enol ether).

Table: Structural properties of major anabolic steroid esters.

Anabolic steroid	Ester				Relative mol. weight	Relative AAS content[b]	Duration[c]
	Position	Moiety	Type	Length[a]			
Boldenone undecylenate	C17β	Undecylenic acid	Straight-chain fatty acid	11	1.58	0.63	Long
Drostanolone propionate	C17β	Propanoic acid	Straight-chain fatty acid	3	1.18	0.84	Short
Metenolone acetate	C17β	Ethanoic acid	Straight-chain fatty acid	2	1.14	0.88	Short
Metenolone enanthate	C17β	Heptanoic acid	Straight-chain fatty acid	7	1.37	0.73	Long
Nandrolone decanoate	C17β	Decanoic acid	Straight-chain fatty acid	10	1.56	0.64	Long
Nandrolone phenylpropionate	C17β	Phenylpropanoic acid	Aromatic fatty acid	– (~6–7)	1.48	0.67	Long
Trenbolone acetate	C17β	Ethanoic acid	Straight-chain fatty acid	2	1.16	0.87	Short
Trenbolone enanthate[d]	C17β	Heptanoic acid	Straight-chain fatty acid	7	1.41	0.71	Long

Butorphanol

Butorphanol is a morphinan-type synthetic agonist–antagonist opioid analgesic developed by Bristol-Myers. Butorphanol is most closely structurally related to levorphanol. Butorphanol is available as the tartrate salt in injectable, tablet, and intranasal spray formulations. The tablet form is only used in dogs, cats and horses due to low bioavailability in humans.

Medical uses

The most common indication for butorphanol is management of migraine using the intranasal spray formulation. It may also be used parenterally for management of moderate-to-severe pain, as a supplement for balanced general anesthesia, and management of pain during labor. Butorphanol is also quite effective at reducing post-operative shivering (owing to its Kappa agonist activity). Butorphanol is more effective in reducing pain in women than in men.

Pharmacology

Butorphanol exhibits partial agonist and antagonist activity at the μ-opioid receptor, as well as partial agonist activity at the κ-opioid receptor (K_i = 2.5 nM; EC_{50} = 57 nM; E_{max} = 57%). Stimulation of these receptors on central nervous system neurons causes an intracellular inhibition of adenylate cyclase, closing of influx membrane calcium channels, and opening of membrane potassium channels. This leads to hyperpolarization of the cell membrane potential and suppression of action potential transmission of ascending pain pathways. Because of its κ-agonist activity, at analgesic doses butorphanol increases pulmonary arterial pressure and cardiac work. Additionally, κ-agonism can cause dysphoria at therapeutic or supertherapeutic doses; this gives butorphanol a lower potential for abuse than other opioid drugs.

Side Effects

As with other opioid analgesics, central nervous system effects (such as sedation, confusion, and dizziness) are considerations with butorphanol. Nausea and vomiting are common. Less common are the gastrointestinal effects of other opioids (mostly constipation). Another side effect experienced by people taking the medication is increased perspiration.

Veterinary use

In veterinary anesthesia, butorphanol (trade name: Torbugesic) is widely used as a sedative and analgesic in dogs, cats and horses. For sedation, it may be combined with tranquilizers such as alpha-2 agonists (medetomidine), benzodiazepines, or acepromazine in dogs, cats and exotic animals. It is frequently combined with xylazine or detomidine in horses.

Butorphanol is frequently used for post-operative and accident-related pain in small mammals such as dogs, cats, ferrets, coatis, raccoons, mongooses, various marsupials, some rodents and perhaps some larger birds, both in the operating suite and as a regular prescription medication for home use, for management of moderate to severe pain.

Although butorphanol is commonly used for pain relief in reptiles, no studies (as of 2014) have conclusively shown that is an effective analgesic in reptiles.

Use in Horses

Butorphanol is a commonly used narcotic for pain relief in horses. It is administered either IM or IV, with its analgesic properties beginning to take effect about 15 minutes after injection and lasting 4 hours. It is also commonly paired with sedatives, such as xylazine and detomidine, to make the horse easier to handle during veterinary procedures.

Side effects specific to horses include sedation, CNS excitement (displayed by head pressing or tossing). Overdosing may result in seizures, falling, salivation, constipation, and muscle twitching. If an overdose occurs, a narcotic antagonist, such as naloxone, may be given. Caution should be used if butorphanol is administered in addition to other narcotics, sedatives, depressants, or anti-histamines as it will cause an additive effect.

Butorphanol can cross the placenta, and it will be present in the milk of lactating mares who are given the drug.

The drug is also prohibited for use in competition by most equestrian organizations, including the FEI, which considers it a class A drug.

Carprofen

Carprofen is a non-steroidal anti-inflammatory drug (NSAID) of the propionic acid class that includes ibuprofen, naproxen, and ketoprofen. Carprofen is the nonproprietary designation for a substituted carbazole, 6-chloro-α-methyl-9H-carbazole-2-acetic acid. The empirical formula is $C_{15}H_{12}ClNO_2$ and the molecular weight 273.72. The chemical structure of Carprofen is:

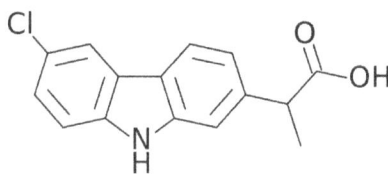

Carprofen is a white, crystalline compound. It is freely soluble in ethanol, but practically insoluble in water at 25°C.

Clinical Pharmacology

Carprofen is a non-narcotic, non-steroidal anti-inflammatory agent with characteristic analgesic and antipyretic activity approximately equipotent to indomethacin in animal models.

The mechanism of action of Carprofen, like that of other NSAIDs, is believed to be associated with the inhibition of cyclooxygenase activity. Two unique cyclooxygenases have been described in mammals. The constitutive cyclooxygenase, COX-1, synthesizes prostaglandins necessary for normal gastrointestinal and renal function. The inducible cyclooxygenase, COX-2, generates prostaglandins involved in inflammation. Inhibition of COX-1 is thought to be associated with gastrointestinal and renal toxicity while inhibition of COX-2 provides anti-inflammatory activity. The specificity of a particular NSAID for COX-2 versus COX-1 may vary from species to species. In an in vitro study using canine cell cultures, Carprofen demonstrated selective inhibition of COX-2 versus COX-1. Clinical relevance of these data has not been shown. Carprofen has also been shown to inhibit the release of several prostaglandins in two inflammatory cell systems: rat polymorphonuclear leukocytes (PMN) and human rheumatoid synovial cells, indicating inhibition of acute (PMN system) and chronic (synovial cell system) inflammatory reactions.

Several studies have demonstrated that Carprofen has modulatory effects on both humoral and cellular immune responses.Data also indicate that Carprofen inhibits the production of osteoclast-activating factor (OAF), PGE$_1$, and PGE$_2$ by its inhibitory effects on prostaglandin biosynthesis.

Based upon comparison with data obtained from intravenous administration, Carprofen is rapidly and nearly completely absorbed (more than 90% bioavailable) when administered orally. Peak blood plasma concentrations are achieved in 1-3 hours after oral administration of 1, 5, and 25 mg/kg to dogs. The mean terminal half-life of Carprofen is approximately 8 hours (range 4.5-9.8 hours) after single oral doses varying from 1-35 mg/kg of body weight. After a 100 mg single intravenous bolus dose, the mean elimination half-life was approximately 11.7 hours in the dog. Carprofen is more than 99% bound to plasma protein and exhibits a very small volume of distribution.

Carprofen is eliminated in the dog primarily by biotransformation in the liver followed by rapid excretion of the resulting metabolites (the ester glucuronide of Carprofen and the ether glucuronides of 2 phenolic metabolites, 7-hydroxy-Carprofen and 8-hydroxy Carprofen) in the feces (70-80%) and urine (10-20%). Some enterohepatic circulation of the drug is observed.

Indications

Carprofen is indicated for the relief of pain and inflammation associated with osteoarthritis and for the control of postoperative pain associated with soft tissue and orthopedic surgeries in dogs.

Contraindications

Carprofen should not be used in dogs exhibiting previous hypersensitivity to Carprofen.

Precautions

As a class, cyclooxygenase inhibitory NSAIDs may be associated with gastrointestinal, renal and hepatic toxicity. Effects may result from decreased prostaglandin production and inhibition of the enzyme cyclooxygenase which is responsible for the formation of prostaglandins from arachidonic acid. When NSAIDs inhibit prostaglandins that cause inflammation they may also inhibit those prostaglandins which maintain normal homeostatic function. These anti-prostaglandin effects may result in clinically significant disease in patients with underlying or pre-existing disease more often than in healthy patients. NSAID therapy could unmask occult disease which has previously been undiagnosed due to the absence of apparent clinical signs. Patients with underlying renal disease for example, may experience exacerbation or decompensation of their renal disease while on NSAID therapy. The use of parenteral fluids during surgery should be considered to reduce the potential risk of renal complications when using NSAIDs perioperatively.

Carprofen is an NSAID, and as with others in that class, adverse reactions may occur with its use. The most frequently reported effects have been gastrointestinal signs. Events involving suspected renal, hematologic, neurologic, dermatologic, and hepatic effects have also been reported. Patients at greatest risk for renal toxicity are those that are dehydrated, on concomitant diuretic therapy, or those with renal, cardiovascular, and/or hepatic dysfunction. Concurrent administration of potentially nephrotoxic drugs should be approached cautiously, with appropriate monitoring. Since NSAIDs possess the potential to induce gastrointestinal ulcerations and/or gastrointestinal perforations, concomitant use of Carprofen and other anti-inflammatory drugs, such as NSAIDs or corticosteroids, should be avoided. If additional pain medication is needed after administration of the total daily dose of Carprofen, a non-NSAID or non-cortico-steroid class of analgesia should be considered. The use of another NSAID is not recommended. Sensitivity to drug-associated adverse reactions varies with the individual patient. Dogs that have experienced adverse reactions from one NSAID may experience adverse reactions from another NSAID. Carprofen treatment was not associated with renal toxicity or gastrointestinal ulceration in well-controlled safety studies of up to ten times the dose in dogs. Carprofen Caplets is not recommended for use in dogs with bleeding disorders (e.g., Von Willebrand's disease), as safety has not been established in dogs with these disorders. The safe use of Carprofen Caplets in animals less than 6 weeks of age, pregnant dogs, dogs used for breeding purposes, or in lactating bitches has not been established. Studies to determine the activity of Carprofen when administered concomitantly with other protein-bound or similarly metabolized drugs have not been conducted.

Drug compatibility should be monitored closely in patients requiring additional therapy. Such drugs commonly used include cardiac, anticonvulsant and behavioral medications. It has been suggested that treatment with Carprofen may reduce the level of inhalant anesthetics needed.

If additional pain medication is warranted after administration of the total daily dose of Carprofen Caplets, alternative analgesia should be considered. The use of another NSAID is not recommended. Consider appropriate washout times when switching from one NSAID to another or when switching from corticosteroid use to NSAID use.

Warnings

Keep out of reach of children. Not for human use. Consult a physician in cases of accidental ingestion by humans. For use in dogs only. Do not use in cats.

All dogs should undergo a thorough history and physical examination before initiation of NSAID therapy. Appropriate laboratory tests to establish hematological and serum biochemical baseline data prior to, and periodically during, administration of any NSAID should be considered. Owners should be advised to observe for signs of potential drug toxicity.

Carprofen Caplets, like other drugs of its class, is not free from adverse reactions. Owners should be advised of the potential for adverse reactions and be informed of the clinical signs associated with drug intolerance. Adverse reactions may include decreased appetite, vomiting, diarrhea, dark or tarry stools, increased water consumption, increased urination, pale gums due to anemia, yellowing of gums, skin or white of the eye due to jaundice, lethargy, incoordination, seizure, or behavioral changes.

Serious adverse reactions associated with this drug class can occur without warning and in rare situations result in death. Owners should be advised to discontinue Carprofen Caplets therapy and contact their veterinarian immediately if signs of intolerance are observed.

The vast majority of patients with drug related adverse reactions have recovered when the signs are recognized, the drug is withdrawn and veterinary care, if appropriate, is initiated. Owners should be advised of the importance of periodic follow up for all dogs during administration of any NSAID.

Adverse Reactions

During investigational studies of osteoarthritis with twice daily administration of 1 mg/lb, no clinically significant adverse reactions were reported. Some clinical signs were observed during field studies (n=297) which were similar for Carprofen caplet- and placebo-treated dogs. Incidences of the following were observed in both groups: vomiting (4%), diarrhea (4%), changes in appetite (3%), lethargy (1.4%), behavioral changes (1 %), and constipation (0.3%). The product vehicle served as control.

There were no serious adverse events reported during clinical field studies with once daily oral administration of 2 mg/lb. The following categories of abnormal health observations were reported. The product vehicle served as control.

Percentage of Dogs with Abnormal Health Observations Reported in Clinical Field Study(2mg/lb once daily)		
Observation	Carprofen (n=129)	Placebo (n=132)
Inappetence	1.6	1.5
Vomiting	3.1	3.8
Diarrhea/Soft stool	3.1	4.5
Behavior change	0.8	0.8
Dermatitis	0.8	0.8
PU/PD	0.8	--
SAP increase	7.8	8.3
ALT increase	5.4	4.5
AST increase	2.3	0.8
BUN increase	3.1	1.5
Bilirubinuria	16.3	12.1
Ketonuria	14.7	9.1

Clinical pathology parameters listed represent reports of increases from pre-treatment values; medical judgment is necessary to determine clinical relevance.

During investigational studies of surgical pain for the caplet formulation, no clinically significant adverse reactions were reported. The product vehicle served as control.

Percentage of Dogs with Abnormal Health Observations Reported in Surgical Pain Field Studies with Caplets (2 mg/lb once daily)		
Observation*	Carprofen (n=148)	Placebo (n=149)
Vomiting	10.1	13.4
Diarrhea/Soft stool	6.1	6.0

Ocular disease	2.7	0
Inappetence	1.4	0
Dermatitis/skin lesion	2.0	1.3
Dysrhythmia	0.7	0
Apnea	1.4	0
Oral/periodontal disease	1.4	0
Pyrexia	0.7	1.3
Urinary tract disease	1.4	1.3
Wound drainage	1.4	0
A single dog may have experienced more than one occurrence of an event		

Post-approval Experience

Although not all adverse reactions are reported, the following adverse reactions are based on voluntary post-approval adverse drug experience reporting. The categories of adverse reactions are listed in decreasing order of frequency by body system.

Gastrointestinal: Vomiting, diarrhea, constipation, inappetence, melena, hematemesis, gastrointestinal ulceration, gastrointestinal bleeding, pancreatitis.

Hepatic: Inappetence, vomiting, jaundice, acute hepatic toxicity, hepatic enzyme elevation, abnormal liver function test(s), hyperbilirubinemia, bilirubinuria, hypoalbuminemia. Approximately one-fourth of hepatic reports were in Labrador Retrievers.

Neurologic: Ataxia, paresis, paralysis, seizures, vestibular signs, disorientation.

Urinary: Hematuria, polyuria, polydipsia, urinary incontinence, urinary tract infection, azotemia, acute renal failure, tubular abnormalities including acute tubular necrosis, renal tubular acidosis, glucosuria.

Behavioral: Sedation, lethargy, hyperactivity, restlessness, aggressiveness.

Hematologic: Immune-mediated hemolytic anemia, immune-mediated thrombocytopenia, blood loss anemia, epistaxis.

Dermatologic: Pruritus, increased shedding, alopecia, pyotraumatic moist dermatitis (hot spots), necrotizing panniculitis/vasculitis, ventral ecchymosis.

Immunologic or hypersensitivity: Facial swelling, hives, erythema.

In rare situations, death has been associated with some of the adverse reactions listed above.

Dosage and Administration

Always provide Client Information Sheet with prescription. Carefully consider the potential benefits and risk of Carprofen and other treatment options before deciding to use Carprofen. Use the lowest effective dose for the shortest duration consistent with individual response. The recommended dosage for oral administration to dogs is 2 mg/lb (4.4 mg/kg) of body weight daily. The total daily dose may be administered as 2 mg/lb of body weight once daily or divided and administered as 1 mg/lb (2.2 mg/kg) twice daily. For the control of postoperative pain, administer approximately 2 hours before the procedure. Caplets are scored and dosage should be calculated in half-caplet increments.

Effectiveness

Confirmation of the effectiveness of Carprofen for the relief of pain and inflammation associated with osteoarthritis and for the control of postoperative pain associated with soft tissue and orthopedic surgeries, was demonstrated in 5 placebo-controlled, masked studies examining the anti-inflammatory and analgesic effectiveness of Carprofen in various breeds of dogs.

Separate placebo-controlled, masked, multicenter field studies confirmed the anti-inflammatory and analgesic effectiveness of Carprofen when dosed at 2 mg/lb once daily or when divided and administered at 1 mg/lb twice daily. In these two field studies, dogs diagnosed with osteoarthritis showed statistically significant overall improvement based on lameness evaluations by the veterinarian and owner observations when administered Carprofen at labeled doses.

Separate placebo-controlled, masked, multicenter field studies confirmed the effectiveness of Carprofen for the control of postoperative pain when, dosed at 2 mg/lb once daily in various breeds of dogs. In these studies, dogs presented for ovariohysterectomy, cruciate repair and aural surgeries were administered Carprofen preoperatively and for a maximum of 3 days (soft tissue) or 4 days (orthopedic) postoperatively. In general, dogs administered Carprofen showed statistically significant improvement in pain scores compared to controls.

Animal Safety Studies

Laboratory studies in unanesthetized dogs and clinical field studies have demonstrated that Carprofen is well tolerated in dogs after oral administration.

In target animal safety studies, Carprofen was administered orally to healthy Beagle dogs at 1, 3, and 5 mg/lb twice daily (1, 3 and 5 times the recommended total daily dose) for 42 consecutive days with no significant adverse reactions. Serum albumin for a single female dog receiving 5 mg/lb twice daily decreased to 2.1 g/dL after 2 weeks of treatment, returned to the pre-treatment value (2.6 g/dL) after 4 weeks of treatment, and was 2.3 g/dL at the final 6-week evaluation. Over the 6-week treatment period, black or bloody stools were observed in 1 dog (1 incident) treated with 1 mg/lb twice daily and in 1 dog (2 incidents) treated with 3 mg/lb twice daily. Redness of the colonic mucosa was observed in 1 male that received 3 mg/lb twice daily.

Two of 8 dogs receiving 10 mg/lb orally twice daily (10 times the recommended total daily dose) for 14 days exhibited hypoalbuminemia. The mean albumin level in the dogs receiving this dose was lower (2.38 g/dL) than each of 2 placebo control groups (2.88 and 2.93 g/dL, respectively). Three incidents of black or bloody stool were observed in 1 dog. Five of 8 dogs exhibited reddened areas of duodenal mucosa on gross pathologic examination. Histologic examination of these areas revealed no evidence of ulceration, but did show minimal congestion of the lamina propria in 2 of the 5 dogs.

In separate safety studies lasting 13 and 52 weeks, respectively, dogs were administered orally up to 11.4 mg/lb/day (5.7 times the recommended total daily dose of 2 mg/lb) of Carprofen. In both studies, the drug was well tolerated clinically by all of the animals. No gross or histologic changes were seen in any of the treated animals. In both studies, dogs receiving the highest doses had average increases in serum L-alanine aminotransferase (ALT) of approximately 20 IU.

In the 52-week study, minor dermatologic changes occurred in dogs in each of the treatment groups but not in the control dogs. The changes were described as slight redness or rash and were diagnosed as non-specific dermatitis. The possibility exists that these mild lesions were treatment related, but no dose relationship was observed.

Clinical field studies were conducted with 549 dogs of different breeds at the recommended oral doses for 14 days (297 dogs were included in a study evaluating 1 mg/lb twice daily and 252 dogs were included in a separate study evaluating 2 mg/lb once daily). In both studies the drug was clinically well tolerated and the incidence of clinical adverse reactions for Carprofen-treated animals was no higher than placebo-treated animals (placebo contained inactive ingredients found in Carprofen caplets). For animals receiving 1 mg/lb twice daily, the mean post-treatment serum ALT values were 11 IU greater and 9 IU less than pre-treatment values for dogs receiving Carprofen and placebo, respectively. Differences were not statistically significant. For animals receiving 2 mg/lb once daily, the mean post-treatment serum ALT values were 4.5 IU greater and 0.9 IU less than pre-treatment values for dogs receiving Carprofen and placebo, respectively. In the latter study, 3 Carprofen-treated dogs developed a 3-fold or greater increase in (ALT) and/or (AST) during the course of therapy. One placebo-treated dog had a greater than 2-fold increase in ALT. None of these animals showed clinical signs associated with the laboratory value changes. Changes in clinical laboratory values (hematology and clinical chemistry) were not considered clinically significant. The 1 mg/lb twice daily course of therapy was repeated as needed at 2-week intervals in 244 dogs, some for as long as 5 years.

Clinical field studies were conducted in 297 dogs of different breeds undergoing orthopedic or soft tissue surgery. Dogs were administered 2 mg/lb of Carprofen caplets two hours prior to surgery then once daily, as needed for 2 days (soft tissue surgery) or 3 days (orthopedic surgery). Carprofen was well tolerated when used in conjunction with a variety of anesthetic-related drugs. The type and severity of abnormal health observations in Carprofen- and placebo-treated animals were approximately equal and few in number. The most frequent abnormal health observation was vomiting and was observed at approximately the same frequency in Carprofen- and placebo-treated animals. Changes in clinicopathologic indices of hematopoetic, renal, hepatic, and clotting function were not clinically significant. The mean post-treatment serum ALT values were 7.3 IU and 2.5 IU less than pre-treatment values for dogs receiving Carprofen and placebo, respectively. The mean post-treatment AST values were 3.1 IU less for dogs receiving Carprofen and 0.2 IU greater for dogs receiving placebo.

Storage

Store at controlled room temperature 15°-30°C (59° - 86°F).

How Supplied

Carprofen Caplets are scored, and contain 25 mg, 75 mg, or 100 mg of Carprofen per caplet. Each caplet size is packaged in bottles containing 30, 60, or 180 caplets.

Xylazine

Xylazine is an analogue of clonidine and an agonist at the α_2 class of adrenergic receptor. It is used for sedation, anesthesia, muscle relaxation, and analgesia in animals such as horses, cattle and other non-human mammals. Veterinarians also use xylazine as an emetic, especially in cats.

In veterinary anesthesia, xylazine is often used in combination with ketamine. It is sold under many brand names worldwide, most notably the Bayer brand name Rompun. It is also marketed as Anased, Sedazine, and Chanazine. The drug interactions vary with different animals.

It has become a drug of abuse, particularly in Puerto Rico, where it is diverted from stocks used by equine veterinarians and used as a cutting agent for heroin.

Medical Uses

Xylazine is often used as a sedative, muscle relaxant, and analgesic. It is frequently used in the treatment of tetanus. Xylazine is very similar to drugs such as phenothiazine, tricyclic antidepressants, and clonidine. As an anesthetic, it is typically used in conjunction with ketamine. Xylazine appears to reduce sensitivity to insulin and glucose uptake in humans. Yohimbine has been used to decrease glucose levels to a healthy level. In clinical settings, Yohimbine can reverse the adverse effects of xylazine if administered intravenously at a dosage of 0.5 mL / 20 pounds shortly after xylazine administration.

Side Effects

Xylazine overdose is usually fatal in humans. Because it is used as a drug adulterant, the symptoms caused by the drugs accompanying xylazine administration vary between individuals.

The most common side effects in humans associated with xylazine administration include bradycardia, respiratory depression, hypotension, transient hypertension secondary to vagus nerve stimulation, and other changes in cardiac output. Xylazine significantly decreases heart rate in animals that are not premedicated with medications that have anticholinergic effects. The decrease in heart rate directly impacts aortic flow. Bradycardia caused by xylazine administration is effectively prevented by administration of atropine or glycopyrrolate. Arrhythmias associated with xylazine includes other symptoms such as sinoatrial block, atrioventricular block, A-V dissociation, and sinus arrhythmia.

Xylazine administration can lead to diabetes mellitus and hyperglycemia. Other possible side effects that can occur are areflexia, asthenia, ataxia, blurred vision, disorientation, dizziness, drowsiness, dysarthria, dysmetria, fainting, hyporeflexia, slurred speech, somnolence, staggering, coma, apnea, shallow breathing, sleepiness, premature ventricular contraction, tachycardia, miosis, and dry mouth. Rarely, hypotonia, dry mouth, urinary incontinence and nonspecific electrocardiographic ST segment changes occur. It has been reported that the duration of symptoms after human overdose is 8 to 72 hours. Further research is necessary to categorize the side effects that occur when xylazine is used in conjunction with heroin and cocaine.

Chronic use is reported to be associated with physical deterioration, dependence, abscesses, and skin ulceration, which can be physically debilitating and painful. Hypertension followed by hypotension, bradycardia, and respiratory depression lower tissue oxygenation in the skin. Thus, chronic use of xylazine can progress the skin oxygenation deficit, leading to severe skin ulceration. Lower skin oxygenation is associated with impaired healing of wounds and a higher chance of infection. The ulcers may have a characteristic odor and ooze pus. In severe cases, amputations must be performed on the affected extremities.

Overdose

The known doses of xylazine that produce toxicity and fatality in humans vary from 40 to 2400 mg. Small doses may produce toxicity and larger doses may be survived with medical assistance. Non-fatal blood or plasma concentration ranges from 0.03 to 4.6 mg/L. In fatalities, the blood concentration of xylazine ranges from trace to 16 mg/L. It is reported that there is no defined safe or fatal concentration of xylazine because of the significant overlap between the non-fatal and postmortem blood concentrations of xylazine.

Currently, there is no specific antidote to treat humans that overdose on xylazine. Hemodialysis has been suggested as a form of treatment, but is usually unfavorable due to the large volume of distribution of xylazine. In addition, due to lack of research in humans, there are no standardized screenings to determine if an overdose has occurred. The detection of xylazine in biological fluids in humans involves various screening methods, such as urine screenings, thin layer chromatography (TLC), gas chromatography mass spectrometry (GC-MS), Remedi HS Bio-Rad Laboratories, and liquid chromatography mass spectrometry (LC-MS).

Multiple drugs have been used as supportive therapeutic intervention such as lidocaine, naloxone, thiamine, lorazepam, vecuronium, etomidate, propofol, tolazoline, yohimbine, atropine, naloxone, orciprenaline, metoclopramide, ranitidine, metoprolol, enoxaparin, flucloxacillin, insulin, and irrigation of both eyes with saline. Effects of xylazine are also reversed by the analeptics 4-aminopyridine, doxapram, and caffeine, which are physiological antagonists to central nervous system depressants. Combining yohimbine and 4-aminopyridine in an effort to antagonize xylazine is superior as compared to the administration of either of these drugs individually due to reduction of recovery time. Research initiatives may be necessary in order to standardize treatment and determine effective measures for identifying chronic xylazine usage and intoxication.

The treatment after xylazine overdose should primarily involve maintaining respiratory function and blood pressure. In cases of intoxication, physicians recommend intravenous fluid infusion, atropine, and hospital observation. Severe cases may require endotracheal intubation, mechanical ventilation, gastric lavage, activated charcoal, bladder catheterization, electrocardiographic (ECG) and hyperglycemia monitoring. Physicians typically recommend which detoxification treatment should be used to manage possible dysfunction involving highly perfused organs, such as the liver and kidney.

Pharmacology

Pharmacodynamics

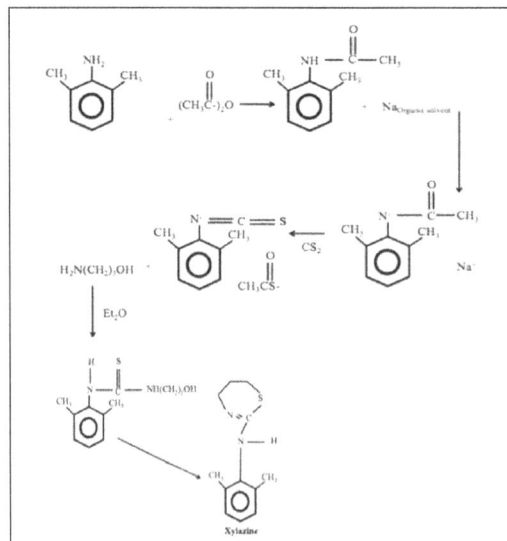

Xylazine Synthesis

Xylazine is a potent α2 adrenergic agonist. When xylazine and other α2 adrenergic receptor agonists are administered, they distribute throughout the body within 30 to 40 minutes. Due to xylazine's highly lipophilic nature, xylazine directly stimulates central α2 receptors as well as peripheral α-adrenoceptors in a variety of tissues. As an agonist, xylazine leads to a decrease in neurotransmission of norepinephrine and dopamine in the central nervous system. It does so by mimicking norepinephrine in binding to presynaptic surface autoreceptors, which leads to feedback inhibition of norepinephrine.

Xylazine also serves as a transport inhibitor by suppressing norepinephrine transport function through competitive inhibition of substrate transport. Accordingly, xylazine significantly increases Km and does not affect Vmax. This likely occurs by direct interaction on an area that overlaps with the antidepressant binding site. For example, xylazine and clonidine suppress uptake of MIBG, a norepinephrine analog, in neuroblastoma cells. Xylazine has varying affinities for cholinergic, serotonergic, dopaminergic, α1 adrenergic, H2 - histaminergic and opiate receptors. Its chemical structure closely resembles the phenothiazines, tricyclic antidepressants, and clonidine.

Pharmacokinetics

Xylazine is absorbed, metabolized, and eliminated rapidly. Xylazine can be inhaled or administered intravenously, intramuscularly, subcutaneously, or orally either by itself or in conjunction with other anesthetics, such as ketamine, barbiturates, chloral hydrate, and halothane in order to provide reliable anesthesia effects. The most common route of administration is injection. The drug is used as a veterinary anesthetic and the recommended dose varies between species.

Xylazine's action can be seen usually 15 to 30 minutes after administration and the sedative effect may continue for 1–2 hours and last up to 4 hours. Once xylazine gains access to the vascular system, it is distributed within the blood, allowing xylazine to perfuse target organs including the heart, lungs, liver, and kidney. In nonfatal cases, the blood plasma concentrations range from 0.03 to 4.6 mg/L. Xylazine diffuses extensively and penetrates the blood brain barrier, as expected due to the uncharged, lipophilic nature of the compound.

Xylazine is metabolized by liver cytochrome P450 enzymes. When it reaches the liver, xylazine is metabolized and proceeds to the kidneys to be excreted as urine. Around 70% of a dose is excreted by urine. Thus, urine can be used in detecting xylazine administration because it contains many metabolites, which are the main targets and products in urine. Within a few hours, xylazine decreases to undetectable levels. Other factors can also significantly impact the pharmacokinetics of xylazine, including sex, nutrition, environmental conditions, and prior diseases.

Xylazine Metabolites		
Xylazine-M (2,6 dimethylaniline)	Xylazine-M (N-thiourea-2,6-dimethylaniline)	Xylazine-M (sulfone-HO-) isomer 2
Xylazine-M (HO-2,6-dimethylaniline isomer 1)	Xylazine-M (HO-2,6-dimethylaniline isomer 2)	Xylazine M (oxo-)
Xylazine-M (HO-) isomer 1	Xylazine-M (HO-) isomer 1 glucuronide	Xylazine-M (HO-) isomer 2
Xylazine-M (HO-) isomer 2 glucuronide	Xylazine-M (HO-oxo-) isomer 1	Xylazine-M (HO-oxo-) isomer 1 glucuronide
Xylazine-M (HO-oxo-) isomer 2	Xylazine-M (HO-oxo-) isomer 2 glucuronide	Xylazine-M (sulfone)
Xylazine-M (sulfone-HO-) isomer 1		

Veterinary use

In animals, xylazine may be administered intramuscularly or intravenously. As a veterinary anesthetic, xylazine is typically only administered once for intended effect before or during surgical procedures.

Side Effects

Side effects in animals include transient hypertension, hypotension, and respiratory depression. Further, the decrease of tissue sensitivity to insulin leads to xylazine-induced hyperglycemia and a reduction of tissue glucose uptake and utilization. The duration of effects in animals lasts up to 4 hours.

Pharmacokinetics

In dogs, sheep, horses and cattle, the half life is very short at only 1.21 to 5.97 minutes. Complete elimination of the half lives can take up to 23.11 minutes in sheep and up to 49.51 minutes in horses. In young rats, the half life is an hour. Xylazine has a large volume of distribution (Vd). The Vd is 1.9-2.5 for horse, cattle, sheep, and dog. Though the peak plasma concentrations are reached in 12–14 minutes in all species, the bioavailability varies between species. The half life depends on the age of the animal, as age is related to prolonged duration of anesthesia and recovery time. Toxicity occurs with repeated administration, given that the metabolic clearance of the drug is usually calculated as 7 to 9 times the half-life, which is 4 to 5 days for the clearance of xylazine.

Detomidine

Detomidine is an imidazole derivative and α_2-adrenergic agonist, used as a large animal sedative, primarily used in horses. It is usually available as the salt detomidine hydrochloride. It is a prescription medication available to veterinarians sold under the trade name Dormosedan.

Properties

Detomidine is a sedative with analgesic properties. α2-adrenergic agonists produce dose-dependent sedative and analgesic effects, mediatated by activation of α2 catecholamine receptors, thus inducing a negative feedback response, reducing production of excitatory neurotransmitters. Due to inhibition of the sympathetic nervous system, detomidine also has cardiac and respiratory effects and an antidiuretic action.

Effects

A profound lethargy and characteristic lowering of the head with reduced sensitivity to environmental stimuli (sound, pain, etc.) are seen with detomidine. A short period of reduced coordination is characteristically followed by immobility and a firm stance with front legs spread. Following administration there is an initial increase in blood pressure, followed by bradycardia and second degree atrioventricular block (this is not pathologic in horses). The horse commonly sweats to excess, especially on the flanks and neck. Other side effects reported include pilo erection (hair standing erect), ataxia, salivation, slight muscle tremors, and (rarely) penile prolapse.

Uses

Sedation and anaesthetic premedication in horses and other large animals, commonly combined with butorphanol for increased analgesia and depth of sedation. In conjunction with ketamine it may also be used for intravenous anaesthesia of short duration.

The drug is normally administered by the intravenous route, and is fastest and most efficient when given intravenously. However, in recalcitrant animals, detomidine may be administered by the intramuscular or sublingual routes. The dose range advised by the manufacturers is 20–40 µg/kg intravenous for moderate sedation, but this dose may need to be higher if given intramuscularly.

When given intravenously, detomidine usually takes effect in 2–5 minutes, and recovery is full within 30–60 minutes. However, this is highly dependent upon the dosage, environment, and the individual animal; some horses are highly resistant to sedation.

Cautions

As detomidine is an arrhythmogenic agent, extreme care should be exercised in horses with cardiac disease, and in the concurrent administration of other arrhythmogenics. The concurrent use of potentiated sulfonamide antibiotics is considered particularly dangerous.

Detomidine is a poor premedication when using ketamine as an anesthetic in horses. Anesthetic recoveries in horses that have received ketamine following a detomidine premedication are often violent with the horse having multiple failures to stand resulting in trauma to itself. Xylazine is a superior premedication with ketamine resulting in safer recoveries.

Atipamezole

Atipamezole is a synthetic α_2 adrenergic receptor antagonist indicated for the reversal of the sedative and analgesic effects of dexmedetomidine and medetomidine in dogs. Its reversal effect works by competing with the sedative for α_2-adrenergic receptors and displacing them. It is mainly used in veterinary medicine, and while it is only licensed for dogs and for intramuscular use, it has been used intravenously, as well as in cats and other animals. There is a low rate of side effects, largely due to atipamezole's high specificity for the α_2-adrenergic receptor. Atipamezole has a very quick onset, usually waking an animal up within 5 to 10 minutes.

Medical uses

Atipamezole is a veterinary drug whose prime purpose is to reverse the effects of the sedative dexmedetomidine (as well as its racemic mixture, medetomidine). It can also be used to reverse the related sedative xylazine. While it reverses both the sedative and analgesic (pain-relieving) effects of dexmedetomidine, atipamezole may not entirely reverse the cardiovascular depression that dexmedetomidine causes.

Atipamezole is licensed in the United States for intramuscular injection (IM) in dogs; it is, however, used off-label in cats, rabbits, and farm animals such as horses and cows, as well as in zoo medicine for reptiles (including tortoises, turtles, and alligators), armadillos, hippopotamuses, giraffes, okapi, and others. It has been given intravenously (IV), subcutaneously, intraperitonealy and, in red-eared sliders, intranasally. IV administration is recommended in emergencies.

Atipamezole has also been used as an antidote for various toxicities in dogs. For example, the anti-tick medication amitraz is commonly ingested by dogs who eat their anti-tick collars. Amitraz works by the same mechanism as dexmedetomidine and is thus easily reversed by atipamezole. Atipamezole also reverses the hypotension caused by tizanidine (a muscle relaxant) toxicity, and relieves toxicity from decongestants such as ephedrine and pseudoephedrine.

Available Forms

Atipamezole is sold at 5 mg/mL for ease of use: 5 times as much atipamezole as medetomidine is needed for full reversal, and because medetomidine is sold as 1 mg/mL, 1 mL of atipamezole reverses 1 mL of medetomidine. When the enantiomerically pure version of medetomidine (dexmedetomidine) was released, it was sold at 0.5 mg/mL, because it was twice as strong as medetomidine. As such, 1 mL of atipamezole also reverses 1 mL of dexmedetomidine.

Specific Populations

Atipamezole is not recommended for animals that are pregnant, lactating, or slated for breeding.

Contraindications

While there are no absolute contraindications to atipamezole, it is recommended against being given with anticholinergics, as both can cause dramatic increases in heart rate. Atipamezole should also not be given too soon after an animal has been given dexmedetomidine mixed with ketamine or telazol(tiletamine); because it reverses only the dexmedetomidine, the ketamine or telazol will still be active, and the animal can wake up excited, delirious, and with muscle contractions. Some recommend not using it in dogs sedated with ketamine at all, since they can convulse due to the excitement effect.

Side Effects

Atipamezole's low rate of side effects is due to its high specificity for α_2-adrenergic receptors; it has very little affinity for α_1-adrenergic receptors and no affinity for most serotonin, muscarinic, and dopamine receptors. There is occasional vomiting, hypersalivation, and diarrhea. It can potentially cause CNS excitement, which can lead to tremors, tachycardia (increased heart rate), and vasodilation. The vasodilation leads to a transient decrease in blood pressure, which (in dogs) increases to normal within 10 minutes. There have been reports of transient hypoxemia. The chance of side effect can be minimized by administering atipamezole slowly.

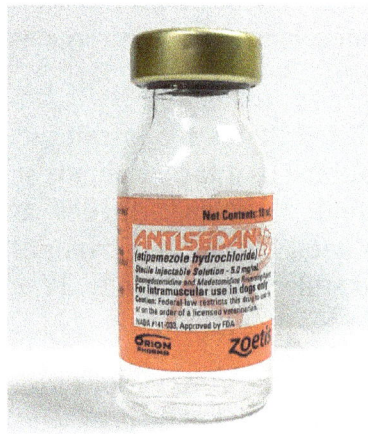

Atipamezole is sold as "Antisedan"

There is a possibility of the sedation reversing abruptly, leading to nervous, aggressive, or delirious dogs. Such cases are more associated with IV administration (which has a faster onset than IM administration). The rapid administration of atipamezole leads to sudden displacement of dexmedetomidine from peripheral α_2-adrenergic receptors; this can cause a sudden drop in blood pressure, which is followed by a reflex tachycardia and hypertension.

There have been some cases where IV administration of atipamezole lead to death via cardiovascular collapse. This is thought to be combination of sudden hypotension added onto the low heart rate caused by sedatives.

There is some possibility of the animal relapsing into sedation after being given atipamezole, made more likely if the original sedative was given IV.

Rats and monkeys have experienced increased sexual activity after being given atipamezole.

Overdose

The LD_{50} of atipamezole for rats is 44 mg/kg when given subcutaneously. The minimum lethal dose in dogs is over $5 mg/m^2$; dogs have tolerated getting ten times the standard dose. Signs of overdose include panting, trembling, vomiting, and diarrhea, as well as increased blood levels of creatinine kinase, aspartate transaminase, and alanine transaminase. Dogs who received atipamezole without first receiving dexmedotomidine have shown no clinical signs other than mild muscle tremors.

Pharmacology

Mechanism of Action

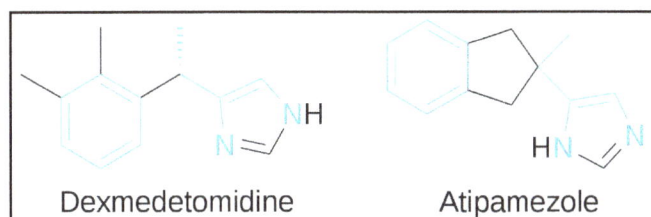

The structures of dexmedetomidine and atipamezole, with the similarities in blue

Atipamezole is a competitive antagonist at a_2-adrenergic receptors that competes with dexmedetomidine, an a_2-adrenergic receptors agonist. It does not directly interact with dexmedetomidine; rather, their structural similarity allows atipamezole to easily compete for receptor binding sites.

Atipamezole reverses analgesia by blocking norepinephrine feedback inhibition on nociceptors.

Pharmacokinetics

Out of the three a_2-antagonists commonly used in veterinary medicine (atipamezole, yohimbine, and tolazine), atipamezole shows the highest preference for a_2- over a_1-receptors, binding to them with a ratio of 8526:1. It shows no preference for a particular a_2-receptor subtype.

Atipamezole has a rapid onset: it reverses the decreased heart rate caused by sedation within three minutes. The animal usually begins waking up within 5–10 minutes. In a study of over 100 dogs, more than half could stand up within 5 minutes, and 96% could stand up within 15. Atipamezole reaches maximum serum concentration within 10 minutes of IM administration. Atipamezole is distributed extensively to the tissues; at a particular time, concentrations in the brain reach two to three times the concentration in the plasma.

Atipamezole undergoes heavy first-pass metabolism in the liver, which includes the glucuronidation at nitrogen during. Metabolites are mostly excreted in the urine.

The elimination half-life is 2.6 hours in dogs and 1.3 hours rats.

Pimobendan

Pimobendan is a relatively new and unique inodilator (inotropic, mixed vasodilator). Its positive inotropic actions are caused by both inhibition of phosphodiesterase III and increased sensitization of myocardial contractile proteins to calcium. Digoxin and other inotropic drugs increase cardiac contractility by increasing the amount of intracellular calcium. Pimobendan improves systolic efficiency without the negative pathway of increasing intracellular calcium. Pimobendan increases cardiac output and reduces both the cardiac preload and afterload. It is usually used in conjunction with other cardiac drugs (furosemide, digoxin, and enalapril). Pimobendan is metabolized by the liver.

Dogs

Pimobendan is used to treat CHF due to atrioventricular valvular disease or DCM. Large clinical-studies support the use of pimobendan in dogs that are symptomatic for CHF and in breeds of dogs that are at risk for the development of CHF due to DCM. The literature is consistently favorable regarding improvement in exercise tolerance, quality of life, and heart failure score. In one study of dogs with CHF due to atrioventricular valvular disease, the dogs that were treated with pimobendan survived 415 days in contrast to a survival time of 128 days for those that were treated with conventional cardiac drugs. The American College of Veterinary Internal Medicine has recommended the use of pimobendan in its 2009 consensus statement regarding the treatment of CHF due to chronic valvular heart disease.

Most animals with clinical CHF will show a rapid response to pimobendan (one week). Cardiac enlargement is generally decreased within 30 days of treatment and the degree of size reduction is correlated with improvement in clinical status and increased survival time. The studies of dogs that are at risk to develop CHF due to DCM have been performed primarily with Doberman Pinschers. The results are strikingly positive with an increased life expectancy of nine months. These studies are being repeated in other breeds..

Side Effects

Side effects that were identified as a part of the field study for FDA approval for Vetmedin® include loss of appetite, lethargy, diarrhea, dyspnea, azotemia, and ataxia.

Precautions

- Pimobendan should not be used for the treatment of hypertrophic cardiomyopathy, aortic stenosis, or any condition where increased cardiac output is inappropriate.

- Pimobendan has been associated with an increased incidence of arrhythmias (both atrial fibrillation and ventricular ectopic beats) but the progression of CHF has also been associated with an increased incidence in arrhythmias. It is not completely understood at this time if the use of pimobendan in animals with CHF is causing an increased incidence of arrhythmia independent of the underlying heart disease.

- Pimobendan has not been tested in pregnant animals, nursing animals or those less than six-months old. It has not been evaluated in dogs with concurrent serious metabolic problems such as diabetes. Not evaluated in dogs with congenital heart defects.

Drug Interactions

Calcium channel blockers and certain beta blockers may decrease the effects of pimobendan.

Overdose

No specific information regarding overdose was found. As a part of the approval process healthy dogs were administered 3X and 5X normal doses for six months without any mortality.

References

- Pedro Ruiz; Eric C. Strain (2011). Lowinson and Ruiz's Substance Abuse: A Comprehensive Textbook. Lippincott Williams & Wilkins. pp. 358–. ISBN 978-1-60547-277-5

- Vaccines-and-vaccination, vaccination-for-animal-health-an-overview, focus-areas: noah.co.uk, Retrieved 14 March, 2019

- Greene, SA; Thurmon, JC (December 1988). "Xylazine--a review of its pharmacology and use in veterinary medicine". Journal of Veterinary Pharmacology and Therapeutics. 11 (4): 295–313. doi:10.1111/j.1365-2885.1988.tb00189.x. PMID 3062194

- How-long-are-rabies-shots-good-3385625: thesprucepets.com, Retrieved 07 July, 2019

- Professional-monographs, acepromazine-maleate-for-veterinary-use, learning-center: wedgewoodpetrx.com, Retrieved 30 May, 2019

- Fornai, F; Blandizzi, C; del Tacca, M (1990). "Central alpha-2 adrenoceptors regulate central and peripheral functions". Pharmacological Research. 22 (5): 541–54. doi:10.1016/S1043-6618(05)80046-5. PMID 2177556

- Duncanson, Graham R. (2012). "Vaccines for sheep. Clostridial diseases". Veterinary Treatment of Sheep and Goats. CABI. p. 97. ISBN 9781780640051.

- Professional-monographs, pimobendan-for-veterinary-use, learning-center: wedgewoodpetrx.com, Retrieved 10 April, 2019

6
Alternative Veterinary Medicine

The use of alternative medicine for the treatment of animals is known as alternative veterinary medicine. A few branches of alternative veterinary medicine are veterinary acupuncture, ethnoveterinary medicine and veterinary chiropractic. The topics elaborated in this chapter will help in gaining a better perspective about these branches of alternative veterinary medicine.

Complementary and alternative veterinary medicine (CAVM) as defined in 2001 by the American Veterinary Medical Association, is "a heterogeneous group of preventive, diagnostic, and therapeutic philosophies and practices. The theoretical bases and techniques of CAVM may diverge from veterinary medicine routinely taught in North American veterinary medical schools or may differ from current scientific knowledge, or both." Although some of the myriad approaches have been used to treat animals for centuries, many have not. Instead, they have been extrapolated from human approaches without first undergoing assessment for safety and effectiveness in nonhuman animals.

Despite the popularity of CAVM among some segments of the public, along with intensive promotion by certain groups, much remains unknown regarding the true therapeutic utility of many aspects of CAVM. Thus, to gain a legitimate foothold in modern medicine, CAVM must demonstrate a rational mechanism of action and withstand scientific scrutiny.

The diversity of approaches that constitute CAM range from the well-studied to the bizarre and baseless. Certain treatments, such as homeopathy, lack biologic plausibility. Others require belief systems more consistent with faith-based healing than medicine. Much of the material published regarding CAM promotes unreliable and potentially dangerous advice. CAM providers cannot always provide a scientific basis and critical perspective for what they practice.

The responsibility for protecting and benefiting veterinary patients remains with the scientifically educated clinician. Veterinarians who consider referring patients for CAVM or practice modalities have a responsibility to distinguish tried-and-true from too-good-to-be-true. This is accomplished by conducting well-designed scientific trials to investigate relevant clinical questions and by regularly reviewing the medical literature to reassess which modalities have accumulated independently confirmed data. Even if a certain clinical application has not yet received research scrutiny, studies showing a plausible and unique mechanism of action, as well as a safety record, can help support a rational decision about whether to recommend it.

Veterinary Acupuncture

Veterinary acupuncture is the pseudoscientific practice of performing acupuncture on animals.

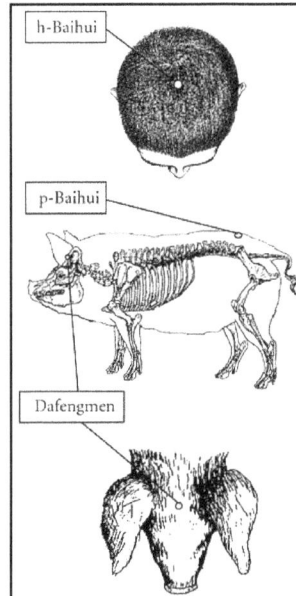

According to traditional chinese medicine, the Baihui acupuncture point in humans, which is the midpoint of a line connecting both ears, is anatomically similar to the Dafengmen point in pigs

Traditional Chinese veterinary medicine (TCVM) has been practiced on animals for thousands of years. For nearly 3,000 years, from the Zhou dynasty and the reign of Emperor Mu around 930 B.C., up until the Yuan dynasty of the 14th century, Chinese medicine was used sparingly on large animals. Much of the focus was on the treatment of horses since they were so essential to the military. In more modern times it has been used increasingly on pet animals. Acupuncture is one of the five branches of TCVM.

In historical Asian culture, people known as "horse priests" commonly used acupuncture. The flow of information from the East to the West regarding animal treatment, including acupuncture, is thought to have started from Mesopotamia around 300 BC. Acupuncture remained a major interest in veterinary medicine for centuries. Its use for dogs was first described in the Tang Dynasty.

In the 20th century, animal acupuncture was first introduced in the United States in 1971 by two acupuncturists of the National Acupuncture Association, Gene Bruno and John Ottaviano. In the process of treating thousands of small animals and several hundred horses, Bruno and Ottaviano trained veterinarians who later founded the International Veterinary Acupuncture Society (IVAS). The demand for veterinary acupuncture has steadily increased since the 1990s.

Practice

Acupuncture is used mainly for functional problems such as those involving noninfectious inflammation, paralysis, or pain. For small animals, acupuncture has been used for treating arthritis, hip dysplasia, lick granuloma, feline asthma, diarrhea, and certain reproductive problems. For larger animals, acupuncture has been used for treating downer cow syndrome, facial nerve paralysis, allergic dermatitis, respiratory problems, nonsurgical colic, and certain reproductive disorders.

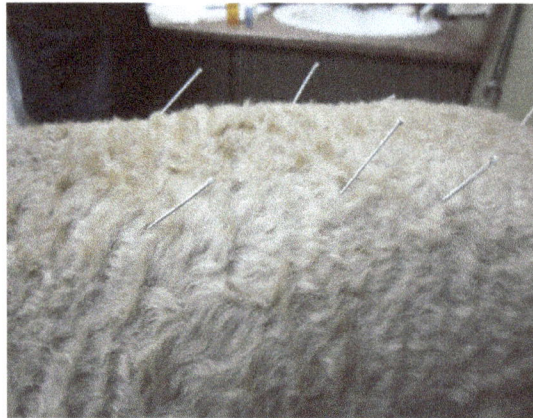

Veterinary acupuncture in dog

Acupuncture has also been used on competitive animals, such as those involved in racing and showing. There are veterinarians who use acupuncture along with herbs to treat muscle injuries in dogs and cats. Veterinarians charge around $85 for each acupuncture session.

Veterinary acupuncture has also recently been used on more exotic animals, such as chimpanzees (Pan troglodytes) and an alligator with scoliosis, though this is still quite rare.

Efficacy

In 2001, a review found insufficient evidence to support equine acupuncture. The review found uniformly negative results in the highest quality studies. In 2006, a systematic review of veterinary acupuncture found "no compelling evidence to recommend or reject acupuncture for any condition in domestic animals", citing trials with, on average, low methodological quality or trials that are in need of independent replication. In 2009, a review on canine arthritis found "weak or no evidence in support of" various treatments, including acupuncture.

David Gorski has said that muscle injuries tend to heal eventually and there is no way to determine if acupuncture had any contribution in the recovery. He said, "For instance, the natural history of most muscle injuries is to heal. They might heal with scarring, so that function is never the same. They might heal and leave the victim with chronic pain. But they do eventually heal."

Related Methods

Acupuncture refers to the use of dry needles; however, there are several related methods which do not use these, or may use a modified type of needle or stimulator.

- Electroacupuncture: Electrical stimulation at an acupuncture point. This may by given on or through the surface of the skin. Various combinations of acupuncture points can be selected to induce electropuncture analgesia in animals. Generally, analgesia is achieved near to the sites of electropuncture.

A study on the use of electroacupuncture on dogs after back surgery reported ambiguous results.

In the study, the post-operation dogs were assigned a pain score eight times within a 72-hour time-frame. Though significantly lower pain scores were found in the treatment group at 36 hours, the scores did not differ from the control group at any other time.

- Aquapuncture: Injection of a drug or a liquid (e.g. vitamin B12) at acupuncture points.

- Acupressure: Application of pressure at acupuncture points.

- Moxibustion: Using a burning herbal stick to stimulate and warm acupuncture points.

- Lasers: Lasers can sometimes be used to stimulate acupunture points.

- Implantation: Gold or silver beads (or other stimulants) are sometimes implanted at acupuncture points.

Ethnoveterinary Medicine

Ethnoveterinary medicine (EVM) considers that traditional practices of veterinary medicine are legitimate and seeks to validate them.Many non-Western traditions of veterinary medicine exist, such as acupuncture and herbal medicine in China, Tibetan veterinary medicine, Ayurveda in India, etc. These traditions have written records that go back thousands of years, for example the Jewish sources in the Old Testament and Talmud and the Sri Lankan 400-year-old palm-leaf frond records of veterinary treatments. Since colonial times scientists had always taken note of indigenous knowledge of animal health and diagnostic skills before implementing their Western-technology projects.

In the 1980s the term "Veterinary Anthropology" was coined for a particular approach to animal health care, which was researched through "using the basic repertoire of anthropology's research skills and techniques, including observation, interview and participation". Ethnoveterinary medicine or ethnoveterinary research was defined by McCorkle in 1995 as:

> The holistic, interdisciplinary study of local knowledge and its associated skills, practices, beliefs, practitioners, and social structures pertaining to the healthcare and healthful husbandry of food, work, and other income-producing animals, always with an eye to practical development applications within livestock production and livelihood systems, and with the ultimate goal of increasing human well-being via increased benefits from stockraising.

Stock owners continue to utilize EVM until better alternatives in terms of efficacy, low cost, availability and ease of administration, are found. By far the most-studied element of EVM is veterinary ethnopharmacopoeia, especially botanicals. Besides, several studies published in recent years have demonstrated the importance of animals as sources of remedies used in medicine for Ethnoveterinary.

Ethnoveterinary and human ethnomedicine practices overlap in several parts of the world. Parallels between medicinal practices in human and animal ethnomedicine not only include the types of resources used and the prevalence of use of those wildlife resources, but also in the modes of administration of these remedies and the ethnomedical techniques employed.

Justification of Studies

According to Tabuti et al. and others, systematic studies on EVM can be justified for three main reasons:

1. they can generate useful information needed to develop livestock healing practices and methods that are suited to the local environment,

2. EVM could be a key veterinary resource and could add useful new drugs to the pharmacopoeia, and

3. EVM can contribute to biodiversity conservation.

Besides, the overlap between natural resources traditionally used as medicines for both humans and animals may be indicative of the efficacy of these remedies.

The importance of gender is being increasingly recognised in EVM. One of the first studies to document gender was conducted by Diana Davis who noted a difference in knowledge of EVM of Afghan Pashtun nomads that paralleled the gender-based division in the society. Davis found that women know more about healthcare for newborns and very sick animals that are taken care of near the home. Since women prepare the carcass for consumption they know twice as many types of internal parasites as men. Women also help with dystocias and the manual removal of ectoparasites.

Another study is that of the Tzotzil Maya shepherdesses who developed their own breed of sheep and have their own husbandry and healthcare system based on their traditions.

In research conducted in Trinidad it was noted that male farmers were using the reproductive knowledge of their female relatives to assist in the health care of their ruminants. Female farmers were using the same plants for their animals that they used for themselves.

ANTHRA, an organization of women veterinary scientists, has been documenting and validating EVM since 1996 in different parts of the states of Andhra Pradesh and Maharashtra in India. ANTHRA chose to study EVM because women farmers performed 50 – 90% of all daily activities related to livestock care but were denied aspects of the local EVM because knowledge was traditionally passed from father to son.

Women are not trained as traditional Dinka healers (atet) in Sudan. However, female-headed households are increasing in Sudan due to war, and women are thus more visible as livestock rearers.

Validation

Herbal remedies used for hundreds of years by stockraisers can be put to commercial use, but scientists are demanding that traditional knowledge should be validated, to verify the safety and efficacy of the treatments.

IT Kenya has a project in the Samburu District that is investigating effective EVM treatments. Vetaid is collaborating with the Animal Disease Research Institute of Dar es Salaam in Tanzania while the Christian Veterinary Mission is investigating EVM in Karamoja, Uganda. Other organizations in the field are ANTHRA and SEVA in India, ITDG and KEPADA in Kenya and World Concern in Uganda. Studies on EVM have been commissioned by UNICEF:

- Wanyama researched and documented information on most confidently used Ethnoveterinary Knowledge among Pastoralists of Samburu, Kenya. The information which was published in a booklet titled "Confidently Used Ethnoveterinary Knowledge among Pastoralists of Samburu" identifies and provides detailed descriptions of top-ten ethnoveterinary practices most confidently used by ethnoveterinary practitioners of Samburu and Turkana communities, in Samburu County, Kenya. The book also attempts to present a methodology that can enable an ethnoveteriary researcher to screen remedies for further scientific trials and value addition.

- Gauthuma tested the efficacy of Myrsine africana, Albizia anthelmintica and Hildebrandtia sepalosa against mixed natural helminthosis in sheep (Haemonchus spp, Trichostrogylus spp and Oesophagostomum spp) in the Samburu district of Kenya. Healers were included in the study and the extracts were prepared following traditional methods including mortar and pestle. Albizia anthelmintica and Hilderbrantia sepalosa treatments showed significant improvement over controls from day 4 after treatment to day 12. On day 12 the three plant remedies showed 100% efficacy while albendazole had an efficacy of 63%.

- Six of the 17 plant extracts used by the Hausa and other tribes of Northern Nigeria for symptoms probably indicative of viral illness were found to have antiviral activity.The extracts of Eugenia uniflora, Acacia artaxacantha, Terminalia ivorensis, T. superba and Alchornea cordifolia showed trypanocidal activity.

- The International Centre of Insect Physiology and Ecology in Kenya is evaluating 40 natural products used against ticks by the Bukusu people in Bungoma District (Wanzala, in process).

- The Onderstepoort Veterinary Institute in South Africa is screening the plants used in EVM for biological activity (Van der Merwe, 2002). Other work in South Africa has been conducted by Masika.

- The anthelmintic efficacies of Teminalia glaucescens (48.4%), Solanum aculeastrum (34.4%), Khaya anthoteca (55.8%) and Vernonia amygdalina (52.4%) were tested by Nfi. Nfi and colleagues had previously tested the insecticidal activity of Nicotiana tabacum and Tephrosia vogelli and plan to test the acaricidal potential of Euphorbia kamerunica and Psorospermum guianensis.

- MacDonald found that the traditional form of usage of Chenopodium ambrosioides infusions as a vermifuge is safer than the use of the herb's essential oil.

- Iqbal compared the in vitro and in vivo anthelmintic activity of *Artemisia brevifolia* with levamisole. In vitro studies revealed anthelmintic effects of crude aqueous (CAE) and methanol extracts (CME) of Artemisia brevifolia (whole plant) on live Haemonchus contortus as evident from their paralysis and/or mortality at 6 h post exposure. For in vivo studies, the whole plant of Artemisia brevifolia was administered as crude powder (CP), CAE and CME at graded doses (1, 2 and 3 g kg(-1) body weight (b.w.) to sheep naturally infected with mixed species of gastrointestinal nematodes. Maximum reduction (67.2%) in eggs per gram of faeces was recorded on day 14 post treatment in sheep treated with Artemisia brevifolia CAE at 3 g kg(-1) b.w. Levamisole produced a 99.2% reduction. However, increase in EPG reduction was noted with an increase in the dose of Artemisia brevifolia administered as CP, CAE and CME.

- Githiori tested seven plant preparations of Hagenia abyssinica, Olea europaea var. africana, Annona squamosa, Ananas comosus, Dodonaea angustifolia, Hildebrandtia sepalosa and Azadirachta indica in 151 lambs infected with 5000 or 3000 L3 Haemonchus contortus in 3 experiments and all were found to be ineffective.

Chinese medicine is also being investigated; treatments historically used for large animals are now being tested on pets. Nagle conducted a randomized, double-blind, placebo-controlled trial of P07P, a product derived from a traditional Chinese herbal remedy. There was a positive result, but it was not statistically significant.

Blanco found that traditional veterinary knowledge of Galicia, northwest Spain was still thriving due to distrust of the veterinary service. However, the traditional system of holding IK as oral knowledge of certain elders is not necessarily a panacea.

The PRELUDE database on traditional veterinary medicine has over 5000 plant-based prescriptions for livestock disorders with each plant listed by family.

Environment, Epidemiology and Health

EVM in future may be increasingly linked to discussions and research on ecosystem health. EVM is now increasingly integrated into "participatory epidemiology" which seeks to improve epidemiological surveillance in remote areas and encourage community participation in disease control. EVM is also studied to provide solutions to diseases in which antigen variation has made vaccination unrealistic and drug resistant strains to Western medicines have become prevalent.

Traditional Chinese Veterinary Medicine

Traditional Chinese veterinary medicine (TCVM) is the ancient veterinary treatment of animals based on the same theories as traditional Chinese medicine (TCM). TCM and TCVM have developed over a period of over 3,500 years and are practiced all over the world. In Western cultures such as the U.S., TCVM has rapidly grown as an adjunct therapeutic modality for animals that do not respond favorably to typical Western veterinary treatments.

Chinese philosophical truths based on Taoism are the underpinnings that influence the practice of TCVM. The fundamental truth for health in TCVM is balance—balance within yourself, balance with others, balance with your diet, and balance with nature.

TCVM practices include four major fundamental branches: Chinese food therapy, acupuncture, herbal therapy,and Tui na ("twee-na").

Its counterpart TCM includes other such treatments as herbal medicine, acupuncture, dietary therapy, and both tui-na and shiatsu massage. Qigong and Taijiquan are also closely associated with TCM.

TCVM has evolved simultaneously with the evolution of TCM. TCVM originated thousands of years ago through meticulous observation of nature, the cosmos, and the human body. Major contributing theories that apply to the practice of both TCM and TCVM include: the Yin-yang theory, the five-element theory, the human body Channel system, Zang-Fu organ physiology, six confirmations, four layers, etc.

Food Therapy

Food therapy is the art and science of combining foods based on their inherent energetic properties. Unlike Western medicine, food is an integral component of treating and preventing disease in TCVM. The Eastern world is focused on the effect food has on the body after it is eaten. Each food item is described as having energetic properties such as warming, cooling, or flavors that act on the body in certain predictable yet different ways. Various food combinations may be used to maintain and support the balance of yin and yang thereby maintaining optimal health. When disease occurs, certain food combinations may be employed to return the body to a balanced state. Food therapy is one of the five fundamental branches of TCVM and a powerful component of the TCVM treatment regime.

Herbal Therapy

Herbal therapy is the use of therapeutic medicines derived from plants, animals, and substances occurring in the natural environment. Herbs are used to move Qi as well as tonify Yin and Yang. Yin and yang are equal yet opposing forces that occur in all naturally occurring phenomena. For instance, Yin corresponds to nighttime, cold, or resting of the body. Yang, on the other hand, corresponds to daytime, heat, and activity of the body. Whenever Yin or Yang becomes deficient or excessive, the balance of the body is lost, and disease results. Herbs are used to restore this natural balance. The Western equivalent to Chinese herbs is pharmaceutical drugs, such as antibiotics and anti-inflammatory medicines. Both western drugs and Chinese herbs are prescribed based on a medical diagnosis. Lately, Western herbals have become popular in the United States. However, distinct differences exist between Western and Chinese herbs. Western herbs are used in a singular form to treat symptoms of disease without a medical diagnosis. Chinese herbs are often a formula or mixture of herbs prescribed according to a medical diagnosis. Generally, in treating a patient, acupuncture is used in conjunction with herbal medicine.

Tui-Na

Tui-Na is medical manipulation with the hands much like the modern versions of Western chiropractic and massage therapy. Various techniques are employed to massage the meridians and enhance the flow of Qi throughout the body. Certified Tui-Na practitioners often teach pet owners several techniques to use at home to enhance the treatment of disease.

Qi-Gong

Qi-Gong is the combination of exercise and meditation in which the flow of Qi is improved. It also is a way to balance the yin and yang of the body. This branch of Traditional Chinese Medicine does not apply to animals.

Veterinary Chiropractic

Animal Chiropractic is a field of animal health care that focuses on the preservation and health of the neuro-musculo-skeletal system. Why? Nerves control everything that happens in your animals. Anything adversely affecting the nervous system will have detrimental effects that will resonate throughout the entire body. The command centers of the nervous system are the brain and spinal cord which are protected by the spine. The spine is a complex framework of bones (vertebra), ligaments, muscles and nerves. If the movement and biomechanics of the vertebra become dysfunctional, they can interfere with the performance of the nerves that are branching off of the spinal cord and going to the all of the muscles and organs. As this occurs, your animal can lose normal mobility; resulting in stiffness, tension, pain and even organ dysfunction. Additionally, when normal movement is affected, and left unattended, it will ultimately impact your animal's entire wellbeing and quality of life.

The nervous system also coordinates the body's ability to heal and regulate itself. Trauma, overuse, or underuse, may cause the vertebra of the spine to become fixed, and the surrounding muscles and ligaments may become compromised and inflamed. Nerves could become trapped in these damaged tissues, or in the passages they use to exit the spine. Their signals become unable to adequately reach their destinations. When they don't, these impaired structures lose their ability to heal. This can directly and dramatically impact your animal's health. Symptoms of spinal fixation are vast, and may include pain, spasm, sensitivity to touch, lameness, gait abnormalities and postural compromise. These are the symptoms that are the easiest to detect. It may take a trained doctor to distinguish some of the more subtle changes that occur when organs begin to malfunction. The goal of an animal chiropractor is to restore function and mobility to the compromised vertebra in an effort to re-establish neurologic transmissions. This allows the body to perform at its optimum potential. These doctors use their hands to identify areas of restriction; and once identified, the animal chiropractor applies a precise thrust on the immobile anatomical structures. This treatment restores the normal motion of the vertebra thus removing neurological interference. When the nerves can efficiently communicate with all the structures in your animals' bodies, they will begin to heal from within. Animal Chiropractic is not meant to replace traditional veterinary care. It is not an alternative treatment, but rather an integrative method that when used in conjunction with good traditional veterinary care, will provide years of happy and healthy living. This is the beginning of a more modern, comprehensive approach to your animal's healthcare. It is an effective and valuable means of restoring and maintaining their strength, vigor and well-being. And by exploring and treating the root causes of your animal's aches, pains and illnesses, will ensure maximum improvement, top performance and an exceptional quality of life for the animal companions we love.

Development of Chiropractic in Animal Healthcare

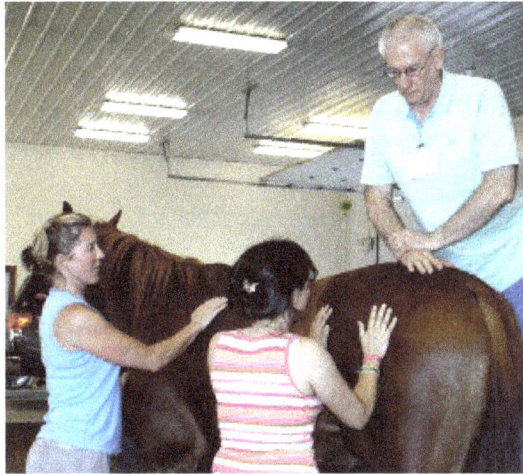

Today, more people recognize that loving and caring for their pets extends beyond providing food and shelter. Quality pet healthcare is no longer limited to spaying and immunizations. With the emerging field of Animal Chiropractic, people are appreciating new ways for their pets to achieve and maintain optimal health. Animal Chiropractic offers non-surgical, drug-free options for correcting bone, disc, and soft-tissue disorders related to improper spinal configuration and movement. When vertebrae become immovable through trauma, injury or degenerative wear and tear, the joints between them become jammed, often affecting the nerves that are in these congested areas. Because the nerves are the communication links from these joints to the brain and spinal cord, messages to the rest of the body become interrupted, leading to pain and loss of function. Animal Chiropractic focuses on the restoration and preservation of heath by removing communication barriers and restoring normal function. This therapy is not limited to an injured or sick pet. Healthy and athletic animals are ideal candidates for chiropractic examination and care. Maintaining proper structural alignment permits optimal function of the muscles, nerves and tissues supporting the joints, resulting in improved movement, stance and flexibility. This alignment promotes increased agility, endurance, and overall performance. Broader benefits include superior immune function, healthier metabolism and a vibrant nervous system, facilitating your animal's natural ability to heal. Chiropractic can enhance the quality of your pet's life, ensuring active and healthy years. More and more often veterinarians are utilizing animal chiropractors in their offices. They do so because animal chiropractors examine and treat areas of biomechanics and the functional nervous system that often go unnoticed by traditional veterinary care. By working in conjunction with veterinarians, animal chiropractors aid in restoring your pet's optimal health by treating the whole patient. Animal Chiropractic is "NOT" intended to assume the primary health care responsibility of animals or replace veterinary medicine.

References

- Management-and-nutrition, overview-of-complementary-and-alternative-veterinary-medicine, complementary-and-alternative-veterinary-medicine: msdvetmanual.com, Retrieved 13 August, 2019

- Sanderson, R.O., Beata, C., Flipo, R.M., Genevois, J.P., Macias, C., Tacke, S., Vezzoni, A. and Innes, J.F. (April 4, 2009). "Systematic review of the management of canine arthritis". Veterinary Record. 164 (14): 418–24. doi:10.1136/vr.164.14.418.

- What-is-animal-chiropractic, animal-owners: optionsforanimals.com, Retrieved 25 April, 2019

- Wanyama, J., 1997. Confidently Used Ethnoveterinary Knowledge Among Pastoralists of Samburu, Kenya Book 1: Methodology and Results and Book 2: Preparations and Administrations. Intermediate Technology Kenya, ISBN 9966-9606-7-8

- Gorski, David. ""Cat-upuncture"? What did those poor cats ever do to deserve this?". ScienceBlogs. Retrieved 17 August, 2019.

Permissions

We would like to thank the editorial team for lending their expertise to make the book truly unique. They have played a crucial role in the development of this book. Without their invaluable contributions this book wouldn't have been possible. They have made vital efforts to compile up to date information on the varied aspects of this subject to make this book a valuable addition to the collection of many professionals and students.

This book was conceptualized with the vision of imparting up-to-date and integrated information in this field. To ensure the same, a matchless editorial board was set up. Every individual on the board went through rigorous rounds of assessment to prove their worth. After which they invested a large part of their time researching and compiling the most relevant data for our readers.

The editorial board has been involved in producing this book since its inception. They have spent rigorous hours researching and exploring the diverse topics which have resulted in the successful publishing of this book. They have passed on their knowledge of decades through this book. To expedite this challenging task, the publisher supported the team at every step. A small team of assistant editors was also appointed to further simplify the editing procedure and attain best results for the readers.

Apart from the editorial board, the designing team has also invested a significant amount of their time in understanding the subject and creating the most relevant covers. They scrutinized every image to scout for the most suitable representation of the subject and create an appropriate cover for the book.

The publishing team has been an ardent support to the editorial, designing and production team. Their endless efforts to recruit the best for this project, has resulted in the accomplishment of this book. They are a veteran in the field of academics and their pool of knowledge is as vast as their experience in printing. Their expertise and guidance has proved useful at every step. Their uncompromising quality standards have made this book an exceptional effort. Their encouragement from time to time has been an inspiration for everyone.

The publisher and the editorial board hope that this book will prove to be a valuable piece of knowledge for students, practitioners and scholars across the globe.

Index

www.ingramcontent.com/pod-product-compliance
Lightning Source LLC
Chambersburg PA
CBHW082036190326
41458CB00010B/3386